Caring for the Living and the Dying

Michael Barbato

To Deanna

Namaste

Michael Barbato

14.11.15

With thanks
to George, Pru
and all my teachers

Caring for the Living and the Dying

Michael Barbato

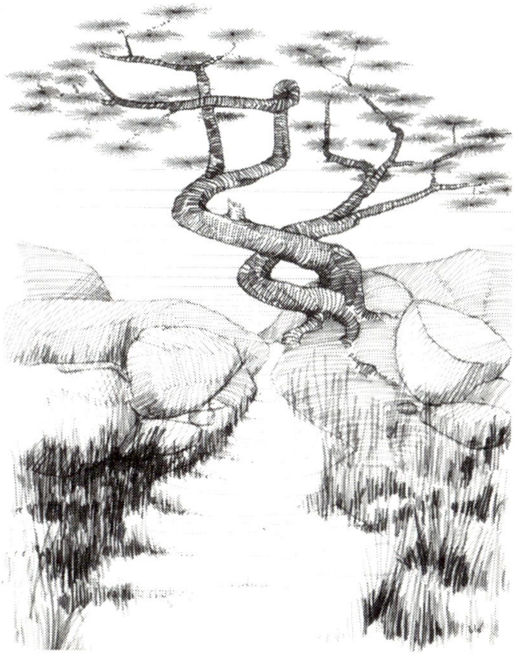

National Library of Australia Cataloguing-in-Publication data:

Barbato, Michael
Caring for the living and the dying

2nd edition

Includes bibliography and index
ISBN 978 0 646 52983 7

1. Terminal care.
2. Terminally ill.
3. Death – Psychological aspects

362.175

Cover drawing: George Ingham

Design (interior and cover): Ruth Barbato

Editor: Jeane Balcombe

Indexer: Michael Barbato

Printed on 70GSM classic by Griffin Press, Adelaide

Other publications by Michael Barbato:
Reflections of a setting sun – healing experiences around death (2009)

Paper used in this book is natural and recyclable, and is made from wood grown in sustainable forests.

Acknowledgments

Almost ten years ago I sat in front of a computer hoping to turn years of palliative care experience into a book that might be of use for those caring for a dying relative or friend. It was a wild idea at the time, but here I am now, completing the finishing touches to a second edition. Palliative care may have changed in the intervening years but not the reason for writing the book. The death of someone you love is one of the most painful experiences you will have to endure. Caring for them as they approach their death is, however, an extraordinary gift that carers can give. It is not an easy task for it is emotionally and physically draining. I hope this book will guide and support those engaged in this wonderful work.

Writing a second edition is a bit like cleaning out the garage – there are some things that need to be discarded, others that are too important to dispense with, and a lot that fall in between. Many people have assisted with this sorting out and tidying up process. Patients and their families have, more than anyone, helped me to see what is important and I am eternally grateful for their guidance and for the teachings they have bestowed upon me. My colleagues, not only the doctors but also the nurses, social workers, pastoral care workers, pharmacists, therapists and volunteers, have refined my understanding of holistic care and have supported me personally and professionally.

I particularly wish to thank my family: Ann, Claire, Ruth, James, David, Rob, Ella and Sol. They are a constant source of inspiration and have helped me to see that anything is possible. I have also capitalised on my daughter Ruth's talents as a graphic designer and I thank her for the skills she has employed and the joy I have felt in having her so intimately involved in the book's production.

I would also like to say thank you to Pru for allowing me to use one of George's drawings for the cover. Finally, to my editor, Jeane Balcombe - thank you seems hardly enough for your guidance, your skills and the gentle way you have directed me in the 'cleaning and tidying up' process. One of the pleasures in writing this book has been to work closely with you. It has been a real delight. *Merci bien.*

Credit. Michael Leunig extracts from the *Common Prayer Collection* by Michael Leunig, HarperCollins Publishers.

Contents

Preface to second edition

Following its introduction into Australia almost 30 years ago, palliative care has grown and matured, and now has a well-deserved and respected place in mainstream medicine. There have, however, been many developments, particularly in the science of palliative care, since *Caring for the Dying* was originally published in 2002, and this has prompted me to produce a second edition.

Once limited to those with cancer and a life expectancy of less than three months, palliative care now has an important role to play in the management of a wide variety of life-limiting illnesses, regardless of life-expectancy. Anyone with a disabling heart, lung, liver or neurological condition can be referred to palliative care for relief of symptoms or end-of-life care. This includes those whose quality of life is undermined by illnesses such as emphysema, heart failure, liver failure, motor neuron disease, stroke, head injury or dementia. Similarly, those who decide to abandon potentially life-preserving treatment such as kidney dialysis or artificial ventilation also come under this broader palliative care umbrella. This more inclusive policy recognises the important contribution palliative care can make to anyone's quality of life, regardless of the underlying illness, its prognosis or the place of care.

This second edition includes updated information on many of the topics covered in the first-edition, and in the Appendix. A new chapter titled *Care of the elderly* looks at the palliation of illnesses other than cancer: namely, heart disease, stroke, dementia, emphysema, leukaemia, lymphoma and kidney failure. It also explores the care of those dying in hospital or nursing homes and of those dying of 'old age'. A separate chapter has been devoted to motor neuron disease because of the special challenges associated with the care of those with this disease. All in all, the second edition is more extensive and covers all the major causes of death within Australia.

Despite mild protests to the contrary, I have kept the word *dying* in the book's title. Many have urged me to avoid the 'D' word, believing it is too confronting and could deter many would be readers. I have not been swayed for I strongly believe the words *death and dying* should be brought into common parlance, otherwise they will always be the proverbial elephant that everyone sees, but no one speaks about. I would like to think my reasoning is sound, but I cannot be certain, for I know that some readers of the first edition carefully hid the cover of the book whenever they opened it in the presence of a sick or dying relative. The new title *Caring for the living and the dying* was chosen partly to overcome this concern, but principally to remind us that those with a life-threatening illness live until they die. It also recognises the important role palliative care plays in supporting those who, after the death of a loved one, must go on living.

As was the case with the original edition, this second edition is written mainly for carers. I hope, however, it will be of value to anyone involved in the delivery of palliative care, as well as to those who have suffered a loss and those who are simply interested in the subject of death and dying.

In 2003, a very dear friend died of cancer. His name was George and I had first met him three years earlier, days after surgery had revealed inoperable cancer of the biliary system. I was asked to see George for pain relief and treatment of his depression. From the moment I sat down beside him, I knew the information I had put together from the medical file did not equate with the person there with me. From the outside he looked no different to many of the hospitalised patients I am asked to see – he was thin, clearly unwell, in some pain, confined to bed and attached to a drip. There was, however, something different. Something I could sense but could not comprehend. It may have been the way he looked at me or the soft and gentle way he spoke and related to me. This man was in pain, but it was not pain that troubled him for, as he lay there, he seemed to be in a state of deep contemplation – almost a meditative state. When I blithely commented, 'you're thinking', he said, 'Yes I am' but offered no more. I felt I was intruding, so resisted the interrogation that often takes place with a first visit.

Gradually we got around to the operation and the cancer diagnosis and at this point, remembering he was 'depressed', I asked a pointed question about how he was feeling. As the words passed my lips I immediately thought – what a stupid question, how do you think he would feel having received a death sentence just days before. George, however, was kinder and did not consider my question inane. Instead, it heralded the beginning of a patient-doctor relationship that went deeper than I had considered possible. His answer was not one I had expected nor was it one I had heard before. He said, I am just considering whether I should die. It was not only what he said but also the seemingly detached way in which he spoke. It took some time before I realised he was not depressed nor was he asking for euthanasia. It was a clean statement of fact.

It turned out that George was a practitioner of *Kyudo* – the essence and practice of ancient Japanese archery. Kyudo is considered the purest of all the martial arts and is practiced as a means of physical, moral and spiritual development. Its aim is not to develop technical expertise but self reflection. This is apparent in the saying of past Japanese masters, who teach that, 'shooting with technique improves the shooting, but shooting with spirit improves the man'. After many years of kyudo, George was able to reflect on his situation in a way that very few of us, myself included, could ever hope to imagine. It was all a question of truth, goodness and grace, the essential principles of kyudo. George was not analysing his situation and deciding what to do, he was reflecting on the how to die gracefully.

Over the next few years George came to visit me many times, sometimes alone and sometimes with Pru, his partner in life. The visits were, in theory, part of the usual medical follow up, but more and more they became spiritual discourses in which I came to know and appreciate George, his way of life and the values he stood for. He was an extraordinary person. Rather than inadequate I felt privileged and blessed to be in his presence, let alone to be his doctor.

George's condition slowly deteriorated. He remained at home until the final few days of his life and died in 2003. He was admitted to the local palliative care unit on a Friday and died the following Monday. I was not present at this time, but Pru said that in his final days, George had many visits from disembodied beings, including one who had been with him after the initial surgery, but had mysteriously vanished after George had been discharged. When George died, Pru felt she traveled with him but at a certain point found she could go no further and suddenly found herself back in her body and by George's now deceased body. She wondered why she did not continue the journey and die with George, but now accepts that her journey was limited by her healthy body, to which she was still connected. She also realised that George's death could not be her death and that hers is yet to come.

Some time after George had died I received copies of drawings he made in the months leading up to his death. Each is a powerful symbolic reminder of his journey from life to death. My favourite, appears on the front cover of this second edition – a book that I dedicate to George, Pru and all my teachers.

Prologue

As a palliative care doctor I am often asked by patients and their relatives how I can do my line of work. There are times when I wonder, too, particularly as many people, doctors and nurses included, are so uncomfortable with death. I suspect the answer lies in the journey my life has taken.

I have clear memories as a young child of accompanying my parents to the homes of their mothers as each was dying, one of stomach cancer, the other of heart disease. I watched them tend my grandmothers and then assist with the ritual washing and dressing after death. I was barely old enough to understand the significance of the occasion, but it was clear, even then, that people we love die. I was overwhelmed to see my parents crying but what struck me most was the amount of love and support such a sad event could summon. The rituals and customs my Italian parents and relatives immersed themselves in suggested that death was no stranger to them. Although unwelcome, it was treated as a part of life and given due respect.

In the following years my family had several uncomfortable brushes with death. My twin sister was run over by a car but miraculously survived unscathed. My eldest brother was involved in a motor vehicle accident in which another person was killed, another brother survived a life-threatening bout of encephalitis and I nearly drowned while swimming in a lake. This was a difficult period for my parents, and at that time it seemed as if our family had cheated death. I believed death had no power over us and, as a young boy I would challenge it to show its face. My bravado appeared to work, for death and its messengers took a break.

It revisited several years later when one of my classmates failed to show at school, another's sister died of leukaemia and another drowned while trying to save children in his charge. These sudden and unexpected deaths were unsettling, but the news that another school friend had killed his mother was incomprehensible. Death revealed a tragic side that I had not previously appreciated. It was not simply a mysterious void that claimed the aged – it respected neither age nor circumstances and could appear unexpectedly. I now feared death and began to exercise caution in what I did.

After graduation in 1966 I began work in a large Sydney hospital where death was an everyday occurrence. At first, I found this overwhelming and emotionally draining, but gradually I learnt not to get involved and became immune to its presence and its devastating effects. This helped me to survive and led to a form of clinical detachment that undermined my ability to empathise with patients and their families.

This approach was severely tested over the ensuing years as five close colleagues died suddenly and at an early age as a result of illness, accident or suicide. Closer to home one of my relatives made two unsuccessful attempts to end his life – on both occasions I found him and initiated resuscitation.

Death had really made its presence known. For the first time I wondered about the meaning of life and the significance of death. I questioned the work I was doing, my motives and what contribution I made to those who were suffering.

Intent on using my recently acquired specialist skills, I moved to a large country town with my young family in tow. In no time I was busier than

I needed to be and only now realise it was because I needed my patients more than they needed me. My sense of self depended on being busy and on what others thought of me. Death was still present but now I saw it as the enemy, an enemy, I mistakenly thought, that could be defeated. I saved many lives, but there were also many who died. My response was simply to try harder.

About this time a young man was admitted to my unit. He'd had a heart attack, but as his condition appeared stable, I reassured him, his wife and their young family that all would be well. How wrong I was. Over the next week his heart stopped numerous times and on each occasion he was brought back to life. I continued to reassure him and his family knowing, deep down, this was false hope. I took it upon myself not to tell them of the danger signs or the distinct possibility of death, even though his and his wife's anxiety was palpable.

The man died and my initial thought was that I'd failed him medically, even though all the important decisions had been guided by specialists from Sydney. It was only when his wife and children stood by their dead husband and father that I realised fear and ambition had clouded my judgment and compromised care. By giving false hope I had deprived them of the chance to say goodbye and prepare for the inevitable. I had abused their trust and failed them in their time of greatest need. I may have been an expert in the care of the body but I had become oblivious and insensitive to the needs of the mind, heart and soul.

Several years of anguish followed as I reached deep within to find some meaning to my life and a reason to continue the work that occupied a large part of it. A change of town and a new job did not provide the answers and only exacerbated the problems I'd hoped to leave behind.

It was around this time that our fourth child, Moira, died unexpectedly of SIDS (cot death) at the age of one month. The effect this had on me and my family cannot be put into words. Moira's death was as incomprehensible as it was tragic, and a large part of us died with her. My wife, Ann, our children and I struggled to come to terms with her death. For my part, several changes of work and two bouts of depression only served to remind me of the despair that had descended on us. The sudden death of Ann's mother, the protracted death of her father from cancer as we cared for him at home, my father's death and the death of several friends rocked our lives even more. Ann and I realised we had to make changes to our life and that I could not continue the work I was doing.

In 1989, fourteen years after Moira's death, we left our beloved country home and our many dear friends and headed for Sydney. To our friends, this was a radical and incomprehensible move, but it was prompted by my decision to start work as a palliative care doctor. I thought I had seen enough death to last a lifetime, but was paradoxically drawn to work beside it.

The twenty years I have since spent in palliative care have provided me with some of my most rewarding and challenging experiences. The work has stretched me to the limit, but being with people as they confront their death is a privilege few have. In some strange and mysterious way they have helped me rediscover a part of myself that was, for some time, lost. This book is a tribute to all those people.

But why write a book about death and dying? It's not a subject most people want to explore; books that deal with this topic usually gather dust on bookshelves and rarely make the bestseller list. So, what is the reason? There are many, but for me the most important motive is to provide family and friends with the knowledge of how best to care for a dying relative. To accompany a dying person on their journey is one of the greatest gifts you can offer and, as with all gifts, the reward is often in the giving.

What dying people fear most is the loneliness that may accompany their dying. The inability to share their fears, anxieties and wishes and to be blatantly honest about their life and death is often more painful than the thought of death itself.

After reading this book, I hope those of you who care for a dying person will be more aware of and able to 'hear' what is in their heart and mind, and less afraid to talk about death. Forty years of caring for the sick and dying has taught me many things, not the least being their need for authentic human contact. Dying is hard, but to die with all one's thoughts and emotions locked inside is tragic.

I would like to thank all those I have cared for and their families. Allowing me to enter into their life at such a vulnerable time has helped me to see the value of trust, love and a life fully lived. I also wish to thank Ann, my partner in life, for being 'nothing less than thee', and our children, whose individual beauty has given Ann and I countless joys and endless rewards. Family, colleagues and friends have sustained me in many ways and I give thanks that they, too, have been part of my journey.

Introduction

I learned that courage was not the absence of fear, but the triumph over it.

NELSON MANDELA
Long Walk to Freedom

Chapter 1

Introduction

Tom was in his mid-sixties and had retired from work less than one year before. He was admitted to the palliative care ward because of breathing difficulties from lung cancer, diagnosed several months earlier. The cancer had not responded to chemotherapy or radiotherapy. When Tom arrived he was gaunt and looked most unwell. I was not surprised when he told me he had come into the ward to die. Such candour is not rare among those confronted with the prospect of dying but what did intrigue me was his refusal to have any treatment to ease his breathlessness. With my medical hat firmly in place I explained how morphine and other treatments could help his breathing and relieve some of the associated suffering. He looked at me, just as my father did when I missed a point he was trying to make. Between breaths, he declared with steely resolve, 'I have heard so much about this dying business, I want to see what it is all about. I want to be awake when it happens and I want to do it well.'

At the time I was surprised by Tom's comment, particularly his request to remain awake. I thought this was unusual, but not his desire to die well. This fundamental hope is as old as civilisation, shown by the many treatises devoted to death and dying. The oldest of these, the Egyptian, Tibetan and Maya Books of the Dead, date back 5000, 1200 and 1100 years respectively. The western equivalent, *Ars Moriendi (The Art of Dying)*, was popular throughout Europe in the fifteenth century and, as with the more ancient texts, emphasised the need to prepare for death.

Given the improvements in medical care, the chances of dying well should be much better now than 500 or even 50 years ago. But that does not seem to be the case. According to Daniel Callahan, 'Death is now harder to predict, more difficult to manage, the source of more and more moral dilemmas and nasty choices, and spiritually more productive of anguish, ambivalence and uncertainty'. Dying may be less painful but the prospect of dying well today remains more of a hope than an expectation. Woody Allen spoke humorously but revealingly when he said, 'It's not that I am afraid of death, I just do not want to be there when it happens'. This deep-seated fear of death is universal and says as much about our unwillingness to forgo life as it does about our fear of the unknown. Death is certainly more of a stranger in the 21st century than it has been at any time in the past.

In wishing that he 'die well' Tom was not asking that his death be 'painless', but that it should be consistent with his wishes and in keeping with the principles that governed his life. A pain-free death was important, but not at the expense of dignity and authenticity. The values he lived by were, not surprisingly, the same values he wished to die by. To do this he needed understanding and respect.

Such courage is not unusual, but is rarely found in those who do not accept the inevitability of death. Acceptance or resignation is the first and most essential step in dying well. Many of us live in fear of death or disregard its very existence. Ironically, it is this failure to integrate death into our life that can make dying such a frightening and overwhelming experience. The paradox is that children and adults see more deaths in one year's TV viewing than any doctor sees in a lifetime of medical practice. Despite or because of this, death has become a matter of fiction rather than of fact – something that only happens to others.

The only thing we can be certain of at birth is that one day we will die. Birth and death are the bookends that hold life together. Rather than deny death, we can instead see it as a beacon that illuminates life, keeps us on course and ultimately guides us home. It helps set our life's course. If we follow this and live with awareness, then death becomes the fulfilment of a life, and not merely its frightening conclusion. Metaphorically speaking, it is the finishing line for the life we have led. We are more likely to finish well if we have run 'the good race'. Living a life that does not acknowledge and respect death can be likened to running life's journey blindfolded.

This book is written to honour those such as Tom who show great courage in the face of death and remain determined not to be defeated by something we all fear yet rarely prepare for. Tom's determination to do it well, even though his fear may have been overwhelming, is unusual and has led me to believe that dying might be easier if people were better prepared for what lay ahead. I wonder why, then, the art of dying well is such a neglected topic. Have you ever thought about what it would be like to die and why death is given so little attention when it is clearly of major importance to all? Fear rather than irrelevancy is what sets the agenda, even when our own death awaits us. The head-in-the-sand approach espoused by Woody Allen does not overcome fear of death; ultimately, dying well will not be possible until the person confronts their fear.

> *Nathan was an imposing figure of a man prior to surgery for bowel cancer. He had been a rebel, and repeatedly defied death by riding a motorcycle fast and furious along many a stretch of road. He lost a leg in the process, but remained defiant and undefeated until the cancer that had slowly eroded his body now started to take over his life. Nathan was frightened, but it was*

hard for a man who had previously feared no person or thing to admit this. Instead, he withdrew to his bedroom or garage and also into himself – it was there, inside his mind, that the real battle took place. As he edged closer to death the fear was almost palpable and it was clear he wanted to talk, but never did. Maybe he did not have the words to tell any of us exactly how he felt.

Then, during one of my routine visits, Nathan asked if he was doing it right. I could almost feel the relief in his voice. While he couldn't talk about his feelings, he could talk about dying as a job that he needed to do and, like Tom, he wanted to do it well. I would like to believe it had parallels with the first time he sat on a motorbike – could he handle it? In his earlier years he would have been too proud and too macho to ask for help, but now he was seeking help and guidance, albeit indirectly, to die well. And he did die well, with a level of courage that exceeded anything he could have believed possible. I had the impression that so much of Nathan's courage had been directed to confronting fear. Only when he openly acknowledged his need for help could he direct this very same courage to dying well.

Death resembles birth in so many ways. Both are processes defined and controlled by nature, and both are accompanied by fear and anticipation. Each journey is different, of varying duration and ends in a transition, one into life and the other into death. While the birth journey is well understood and divided into known stages, the death journey is less clearly demarcated but nonetheless has its own stages of labour. In western society, many birth and death journeys are made within a hospital, but increasingly, there is a move away from this clinical environment into the home.

Birth and death are the bookends of life.

MERRILL COLLETT
At Home with Dying

Whatever the setting, every journey is made alone, but each is assisted and sometimes made possible by the actions of an intermediary. This is where the parallels stop. Birthing classes prepare mothers for what lies ahead and highly skilled midwives ensure, as far as is possible, a safe natural birth. There are, however no dying classes and few people, including doctors, are skilled in the art of facilitating a safe and natural death. This was not always the case: in years past parents and extended family not only acted as midwives at birth but frequently delivered their dying child or other family member into death. This is still the case in many poorer countries but, in Australia and other developed countries, men and women in white coats preside over the death as relatives and friends of the dying sit by helplessly, watching something they do not fully understand.

As with Tom, dying may be natural and medication free. That, however, is the exception rather than the rule. Very few people now die without treatment for some form of physical, psychological or spiritual pain. While most of this treatment is initiated by health care workers, its implementation frequently falls to the carer who, in essence, acts as the midwife. This midwife, unlike her birthing counterpart, is inexperienced, but will be called upon to make decisions and carry out procedures that are unfamiliar and onerous. The aim of this book is to give carers greater insight into the wider dimensions of the dying process and help each one become a skilled midwife as they care for their dying loved one.

This book addresses many of the questions families have put to me over the years. Most common were those related to physical care and comfort as well as practical day-to-day matters. People were hungry for knowledge, for they wanted to deliver the best care possible and needed to know they were doing the right thing. Consequently, much of the material within this book relates to physical comfort, but as physical comfort cannot be separated from emotional and spiritual issues, a holistic approach is taken on most matters. Originally, the book was written particularly, but not exclusively with cancer in mind. In keeping with developments in palliative care, however, this newly revised second edition includes updated material in most chapters together with a new chapter on the palliation of other life-limiting illnesses such as cardiac failure, strokes, head injuries, kidney failure, lung disease and dementia.

Whatever your reasons for reading *Caring for the living and the dying,* I hope you will find something of value within that gives you strength and a measure of reassurance while continuing that most privileged of all tasks – journeying with a fellow human being as they die.

This book is not meant to glamorise death. Loss of life comes at an unimaginable and immeasurable cost. Pain and grief are inescapable and the strength required to complete the task of caring is enormous. It is almost as great for family and friends as for the dying person. Grahame Jones, in his book *Magnanimous Despair*, says, 'The strength I need to die is nothing compared to that which will be required of those who must go on living'. And so it is. Death spells the end of pain for the one that dies but heralds a new and surreal form of living for those that remain. Death is a momentous time in any person's life. Bearing this in mind, the book discusses some of the ways your loved one's dying may affect you and how you can care for yourself as you continue this most loving of all tasks.

Recognising that we care for people, not patients, I have tried to avoid the use of the impersonal 'patient'. This was unavoidable at times, and I apologise for when the personal was sacrificed for the sake of clarity. The terms 'palliative care unit' and 'hospice' are used interchangeably throughout the book. All case reports are true but names, other than Steve's, have been changed to try to ensure anonymity. Steve asked that his name be used if ever I wrote about him.

The strong are here to look after the weak, son,
and the weak are here to teach the strong.

TIM WINTON
Cloudstreet

Chapter 2

Palliative care

At the heart of modern medicine
is a conflict about the place and meaning
of death in human life.

DANIEL CALLAHAN

Chapter 2

Palliative care

Once the natural and expected consequence of illness, death is now considered to be the enemy and, within the hospital situation, it is often recorded as an adverse event and becomes the subject of much soul searching and clinical review. Not surprisingly then, the purpose of most treatments is to effect cure, but if this is not possible the goal shifts to prolonging life. This is especially true of cancer, where first line treatment is usually followed by less effective and often more toxic alternatives in the hope that a cure will ultimately result or, failing that, death will at least be deferred. In this setting, modern medicine struggles to reconcile the value of human life with the place and meaning of death. Does it continue to offer successive treatments, even when the potential for improvement diminishes and toxicity increases, or does it adopt a more holistic approach to care? Does it place any value on the need to prepare for death?

Until quite recently, those dying of a prolonged illness were anomalies in a health system that was focussed on cure. It appeared that medicine had little if anything to offer when cure was no longer possible, and those who 'failed to respond' often became casualties within a system that regarded death as a failure of treatment. Medicine has conquered many diseases but it did overlook two indisputable facts – it will never conquer death, and a peaceful death is as important as the pursuit of a cure.

Drs Elisabeth Kübler-Ross and Dame Cicely Saunders had long recognised the importance of a peaceful death and in 1967 Dame Cicely Saunders created a model of care that sought to address the unmet needs of those who were dying. This form of care is called palliative or hospice care, and has gradually, over recent years, been accepted within mainstream medicine. Apart from benefiting those living with a life-limiting illness it has also led traditional medicine to re-evaluate its attitude and practice towards the care of the dying.

The palliative care model has grown and spread worldwide, but just as medicine has changed, so too has palliative care. In its formative years, people dying of cancer were its sole beneficiaries. The model we have today is more inclusive and offers care to those with diseases other than cancer as well as to people whose disease is not necessarily terminal and for whom quality of life is as important as length of life. Palliative care has not only resulted in better and more holistic care of those with an 'incurable' illness, but has also slowly awakened the health care profession and society to the significance of death and the importance of caring for those who are dying.

Palliative care has been an integral part of the Australian health care system for almost forty years, and services now exist in all capital and most regional centres. Despite this, confusion still exists in the mind of the public and also within the health care profession as to what palliative care is, what it does and how it interfaces with other medical services. Care of the dying is complex and challenging enough without the added confusion of deciding who you can call upon in time of need. If you are new to the caring role you will have had little exposure to palliative care. The following information is therefore offered to maximise your ability to care for the one you love. Palliative care cannot prevent death but, as Callahan says, it, 'changes the way people are cared for at the end of life and substantially reduces the burden of illness'.

What is palliative care?

Palliative care is a philosophy as much as a practice. It sets out to improve the quality of life of those with a life-threatening illness so they can live as full and active a life as their situation allows. The core values as set out by Palliative Care Australia are as follows:

- Palliative care is the active total care of people whose disease is not responsive to treatment. Care is delivered by coordinated medical, nursing and allied health services that are provided, where possible, in the environment of the person's choice. Control of pain and of other symptoms, and of psychological, social, emotional and spiritual problems is paramount.
- The goal of palliative care is the achievement of the best possible quality of life for patients and their families and friends. Many aspects of palliative care are also applicable earlier in the course of the illness in conjunction with treatment aimed at cure.

Who provides palliative care?

Palliative care is delivered by a team of people. The most important person, by far, is the one who provides day-to-day care, usually an immediate family member. Relatives, friends, the general practitioner (GP) and community nurses are also vital members of this team and are the ones most likely to be called upon in times of need. GPs are ideally placed to do much of the medical work as they have the appropriate medical knowledge and are in regular contact with other specialists. They know the family and are more familiar with significant details and family dynamics that could influence care or complicate grief. Nurses are available to help with physical care. They monitor day-to-day progress and assess your loved one's response to treatment. They can answer your questions and liaise with the GP or other members of the palliative care team. Relatives and friends offer physical and moral support and can be relied upon when the going gets tough.

You may be surprised to learn that carers feature so high in the list of providers, but in the home they oversee all the care and deliver much of it themselves. They not only fulfil a vital role in ensuring that pain and other symptoms are controlled, but are also the patient's main source of emotional comfort.

Other members of the team include specialist palliative care nurses and doctors, social workers, the counsellor, physiotherapist, occupational therapist, and pastoral care worker, and numerous volunteers. These people are available to help resolve problems, supply equipment (such as oxygen concentrators, hospital beds and commodes) or provide essential back-up for the GP. Referral to a palliative care team automatically carries with it access to any or all team members. The referral is usually made by the GP if the person is at home, or by a hospital specialist if the person is in hospital. Contact details for the nearest palliative care service can be obtained from your state or territory association (see Appendix).

A special mention should be made of the enormous contribution volunteers make to palliative care and how they can assist carers. Volunteers come from all walks of life and bring with them their own life skills and experiences. Many have been carers in the past and are therefore well attuned to the difficulties of caring for a loved one. Volunteers participate in a special training program that defines their role and responsibility and prepares them for the emotional and physical challenges they may encounter. To find out more, contact your nearest palliative care service and ask to speak to the volunteer coordinator. He or she will tell you about the service and what it can offer.

Here are a few of the ways volunteers can assist you at home.

- **Day respite.** This provides you with an opportunity to shop, visit friends or attend to business, knowing a responsible and skilled person is attending to your loved one's needs or simply being a companion to them. Day respite usually takes place in your home but is sometimes available in specialised palliative care day centres. The latter occasionally offer transport to and from the centre if that is required.

- **Night respite.** Some but not all volunteer services offer night respite, which is useful if you have had a few rough nights and are short on sleep. A volunteer stays overnight and attends to problems that may arise while you catch up on sleep.
- **Companionship** for you and your loved one, particularly if you are socially or geographically isolated.
- **Transport** to and from appointments if no other means of travel is available or practical.

Is palliative care only for those close to death?

In its early years palliative care was almost exclusively concerned with the care of those who were close to death. Most were treated within hospices and very few returned home. Palliative care was therefore seen as terminal care and referral carried with it the understanding that death was near. In keeping with this, people were accepted for palliative care only if they had a life expectancy of less than three months.

Those days have long gone and referral to palliative care no longer depends on proximity to death. Contemporary palliative care focuses on quality of life and symptom control, and this can be as important in the earlier stages of a life-threatening disease as it is around the time of death. That is not to say care of people at the end of life is given a lesser status. The importance of a good death is still an integral part of palliative care, but it is now part of a continuum of care and assumes increasing importance as a person's health deteriorates.

Consequently, early rather than late referral to palliative care is standard rather than exceptional. It is not uncommon now for those with cancer, heart, lung, kidney and liver disease, motor neuron disease or stroke to receive specific and life-prolonging treatment at the same time as their palliative treatment. This may appear contradictory but a two-pronged approach makes a lot of sense. Specific treatment targets the disease while palliative care attends to symptoms that undermine that person's quality of life. This approach to care is now very common for many life-limiting illnesses.

Unfortunately, the old and now mistaken view that palliative care is only for the dying has led many of those with a life-threatening disease, or their family, to decline palliation when it is first offered. Comments like, 'I did not know I was that sick' or 'it will frighten Mum (or Dad)' are not unusual, and indicate a disturbing misunderstanding of contemporary palliative care. The irony is that people are almost certainly already receiving some form of palliative care at the time of referral, and what the referring doctor wants is specialist advice, not a new approach to care.

In reality, the fear is not to do with palliative care or what it has to offer, but with what it signifies. The association between palliative care and death is so firmly entrenched that many people believe that in accepting it they are 'giving up'. Nothing could be further from the truth. The goals of disease-specific treatment and palliative care are similar – they both aim for an improved quality of life. The only difference is that they operate on different fronts. One takes a curative or disease-modifying approach, the other adopts a more holistic or person-specific model of care. These goals are not mutually incompatible but mutually beneficial.

My hope is that the health profession and the community will ultimately see palliative care for what it is – a form of care specific to the person rather than the disease; care that bears no temporal relationship to death and where the goal is the achievement of the best possible quality of life. The purpose of palliative care is to help any person with a life-threatening illness to live as full and active a life as possible; only when life is clearly drawing to an end does the intent change to facilitating a dignified death.

How it achieves these goals varies from individual to individual. For most it means symptom control – relief of pain, breathlessness, nausea or whatever. In some cases this may be all, but for others, psychological, family, spiritual or existential issues may be equally disabling and require attention. No doctor or nurse has the skills to deal single-handedly with the full range of challenges that may arise, and other members of the palliative care team are frequently called upon to assist. If the problem is pain, a palliative care doctor will be consulted; if it is fear or depression, then a counsellor or social worker is better qualified to advise.

As death approaches, palliative care maintains the emphasis on comfort and seeks also to facilitate a dignified death in the dying person's place of choice. It helps with day-to-day care, fine tunes medication, supports the family and friends and keeps them informed, as much as is possible, on changes, developments and treatment options. This can be a tense and uncertain time and the daily and often twice daily visits by the doctor and/or nurse can be reassuring and empowering.

Who is eligible for palliative care?

Palliative care was established to deal with the specific and often neglected problems experienced by those with advanced or incurable cancer. In time, cancer patients with less advanced forms of the disease but with equally troublesome symptoms were included and now people with a whole range of illnesses come under the palliative care umbrella. These illnesses include AIDS, lymphoma, leukaemia, motor neurone disease, emphysema, intractable heart problems, liver failure, and renal failure where dialysis or transplantation is not possible or is declined.

The only requirements that need to be met for a palliative care referral are:

- a progressive illness that is beyond cure or where there is no known cure
- symptoms, both physical and psycho/spiritual, that are distressing or compromise a person's quality of life
- the consent of the patient and/or family for the referral to be made.

Are children eligible to receive palliative care?

There is no upper or lower age limit for people requiring palliative care. Children do, however, present special challenges that are best met by the treating paediatric team. They have the necessary expertise to provide excellent palliation and are known and trusted by the child and his/her family. Most paediatric palliative care takes place within the home or a hospital-based paediatric unit. Only a few large centres have dedicated paediatric palliative care units to provide much needed respite for parents and family as they care for a chronically sick or dying child. Information on these units is obtainable through state and territory associations or the paediatric service that cares for the child.

Can palliative care be given at home?

Contrary to popular belief, most palliative care is delivered in a person's home. This is not to say most of these people die at home, but that many of the problems experienced by the person can be adequately managed at home. In fact, only 15 per cent of people receiving palliative care die in their own home; the majority die within a hospital (60 per cent) and the remainder in a palliative care unit or nursing home. Although the number of home deaths has not increased over the years, the length of time a person spends in hospital or a hospice during their last year of life has been substantially reduced because of palliative care.

A home death is possible and in many cases desirable, but social and/or medical problems often make this difficult. Care and comfort is not compromised with a home death unless there are complex or testing medical problems, and then hospice admission is recommended. Two other common impediments to a person dying at home are carer exhaustion and a family's fear of inadequacy in the face of a crisis. In either case, it is usually better all round for admission to be arranged.

When and why are people admitted to a palliative care unit?

Palliative care units are present in most urban and regional centres. If there is no such unit, the local hospital usually has one or more dedicated palliative care beds and prioritises them for palliative care patients who require admission. Hospitals may or may not have a specialist palliative care team, but they do have knowledge of palliative care principles and will, when necessary, contact the nearest regional service for advice.

Whether it is a hospice or hospital, admission is usually for one of the following reasons.

- **Symptom control.** If a symptom does not respond to treatment at home or if the symptom is too distressing, admission to a specialised palliative care unit is often the best way to achieve rapid relief. Once this is achieved, discharge to home usually follows. The length of stay will naturally depend on the nature and severity of the problem.
- **Respite care.** A respite admission is a pre-planned admission with the expressed purpose of giving the carer a break. The duration may be as short as one day or as long as two weeks, depending on the circumstances. During this time the unit provides ongoing care while the carer catches up on much needed rest, has a well-earned break or attends to other matters. Respite admissions need to be booked in advance and, given the heavy demand for palliative care beds, are always subject to a bed being available at the time. Patients requiring symptom control or end-of-life care are always given priority.
- **End-of-life care.** This is for people who cannot be cared for at home during the final days or weeks of life.

There is no limit to the number of times a person can be admitted for symptom control and respite care. A minimum interval of six to eight weeks or thereabouts is, however, usually imposed between each respite admission.

Quite often it is not the availability of beds but emotional factors that delay or stand in the way of a much needed admission. Your loved one may be afraid they will not see home again or you, the carer, may be overwhelmed by guilt, fear or anxiety, and so resist the admission. These feelings are absolutely normal but should be carefully weighed against the reason for admission and the possible consequences of delay. If this is the case, a satisfactory compromise is often possible after a full and honest discussion. I have found most people are prepared to follow a reasonable recommendation provided they hear the reasons for it and are given the opportunity to air their concern(s).

Another reason why carers resist admission is the promise they may have made to their loved one, often long ago, to continue care at home. Carers feel duty bound to honour this and can be burdened by guilt if admission to a palliative care unit or hospital becomes necessary. It goes without saying that the course of a life-threatening illness is unpredictable and, despite the best intentions, there are times when the burden of care becomes too great. For this reason, a blanket promise to continue care at home is best avoided. A conditional promise that care will continue as long as it is humanly possible and medically reasonable is one that most people understand and accept.

Carer fatigue is a common problem and can be a reason for a planned or urgent admission. If you have reached a point where you can no longer continue, whether for physical or emotional reasons, it is in your and your loved one's interests to acknowledge the need for help. Be very open about your concerns, share them with your loved one and discuss them with the doctor or nurse. You may feel as though you have let your loved one down but, remember, we all have our limits. So do not punish yourself. Recognise the enormous commitment you have already made. The need for admission can arise despite the best efforts of you and the palliative care team. The exhaustion factor is very real. Ann and I looked after a dying relative at home for six weeks as he was dying of cancer. Despite our respective nursing and medical backgrounds we struggled, and often felt inadequate or unable to carry out the numerous tasks required of us.

If possible, I recommend that you visit the nearest palliative care unit or hospital. Seeing the unit and talking to staff usually dispels most but not all the fear, and allays much of the anxiety associated with an admission.

It is desirable to take your sick relative with you but, if that is not possible, they should at least be informed about the visit and your impressions.

There may be reasons why you prefer your loved one to be admitted to a hospital rather than a palliative care unit. This is particularly true for those who have a long association with one specialist and his/her ward. The reassurance that comes with familiar surroundings and personnel is recognised and the palliative care team can, if you prefer, arrange a hospital admission. Once again, bed availability may be a factor in the final choice. Without trying to influence the decision, I feel obliged to speak up in favour of the hospice option. When compared to hospitals they are less busy, more homely, have fewer restrictions and are better positioned to care for everyone's needs. These may or may not be important for the patient (or family), but what does seem to matter is that admission to a hospice bed is direct. If, however, the patient chooses to go to hospital, they are, almost always, admitted via the Emergency Department, with all the associated delays and discomforts.

How does a palliative care unit differ from a hospital?

A palliative care unit is not, as many people suspect, a private hospital. It is part of the general hospital system funded by the state or territory government. The unit may be located within a general hospital or in a separate building within or outside the hospital grounds. It tends to be smaller, quieter, less hectic and less clinical than the average hospital ward. It has fewer restrictions, hardly any machines, no intravenous drips and none of the usual interruptions such as regular blood pressure or temperature readings. Families, but rarely patients, are often surprised by this, particularly if their relative has come from or spent a considerable time within a general hospital.

For some of those used to the hustle and bustle of a hospital, this low-key approach may be regarded as unusually casual. This may be so, but let me assure you, this does not mean care is compromised. Quite the opposite! Palliative care strives for a homely approach and, just as care is not compromised at home by the absence of blood pressure or temperature readings, so too within the palliative care unit. Of course, there are times when tests or procedures are necessary – when this is the case palliative care units have the necessary facilities and the expertise.

You may wonder how a person's condition can be monitored when tests and 'vital signs' are not checked regularly. The truth is, these observations are of very little value in the palliative care situation and rarely tell us anything we don't already know. More importantly, no amount of testing will tell us about a person's emotional or spiritual well-being – yet it is these areas, rather than the person's physical status, that are most in need of monitoring. Sitting on the edge of the bed, listening to what is being said, is much more valuable than any measurement and gives more information than any investigation. Staff in a palliative care unit may not be engaged in checking 'vital signs' but they are highly focused and attuned to what may be vital for the person occupying the bed.

Another common misconception is that a palliative care unit is full of people who are dying, and is therefore a depressing place for both patients and visitors. There are many sick patients in any palliative care unit, but no more than in any hospital ward. Most are admitted for symptom control and the majority of these are discharged home. Whenever possible, those who are dying are cared for in the privacy of a single room. Surprisingly, it is not the patients who are concerned about deaths in the unit but their relatives. Many of those admitted have, by this stage, come to terms with the inevitability of death and are not surprised or alarmed when another patient dies.

As palliative care units are part of the public hospital system there is no financial cost to patients, provided they are admitted as 'hospital' patients. Those with private health insurance may choose to be admitted as a private patient, but this carries no added privileges such as a single room or the choice of doctor. Specialist palliative care doctors, nurses, volunteers and members of the allied health team who work in that unit provide all the necessary care. Your GP or previous specialists will not be able to manage your case but can visit and, any recommendations they make will always be welcomed.

Many, but not all palliative care units in Australia have some links with the Christian faith. Usually there are no visible signs to indicate this other than a chapel or a 'quiet room' that functions as a non-denominational place of silence and worship. People of all faiths and those with no formal religious or spiritual beliefs are admitted and can rest assured there is no proselytising or attempts at conversion. Patients may ask their own minister, priest, rabbi, monk or imam to visit and are encouraged to continue their own spiritual practices and rituals.

Is a palliative care unit depressing?

This is one of the commonest concerns people have about palliative care units. It is not an unreasonable inquiry but, in reality, the question carries with it many of the inquirer's own feelings about the nature of the work and about death itself. It says as much about their pain as it does about their perception of palliative care.

I have found working in palliative care challenging but extremely rewarding, not only because of what can be done but also because of what I have learnt and continue to learn. But it was not always like this. For three years as a student and a further three years as a doctor I worked in a large Sydney hospital that had its own hospice less than 100 metres away. In all those years I never once visited that hospice or the people within. It seemed a forbidding place and excuses not to visit came easily. I had been trained to save lives and knew those admitted to 'that place' were dying. I would console myself and justify my absence with the belief there was nothing I could do to help. That was how I rationalised my actions but, if the truth be known, the thought of confronting death on such a large scale was more than I could handle at the time. Like Woody Allen, I preferred to be as far removed from death as possible.

Ironically, I returned to Sydney twenty years later as Medical Director of that same hospice. Much to my surprise and delight the hospice was neither dark nor depressing and the people, although unwell, were more focused on living than many of my 'well' friends. There were certainly times of darkness but, as with nature, brilliant sunshine and rainbows often followed the darkest moments. It had taken twenty years but, true to TS Eliot's words, I now knew the place for the first time.

So, no, a palliative care unit is not so depressing, but it is not a place for the faint-hearted. I tell doctors who are considering a move into palliative care not even to consider the move unless they are prepared to be challenged and to grow. Working at the front line with dying people will shake any preconceived ideas about life and death. As a carer and someone very close to the person who is dying, you too will be challenged and often these challenges may seem insurmountable. But just as dawn always follows night, any darkness you experience will ultimately lift.

One thing that initially surprised me and continues to surprise others is the amount of humour that comes from the lips of those who are dying. This may surface in general conversation, during times of reminiscing or as they talk about the future. It may occur as they luxuriate in a spa bath or relax during a foot massage. Much of the humour is dark but it is liberating and gives sick people the opportunity to talk about important things in a lighter vein. There have been times when I did not know whether to laugh or cry. Here are a few examples of their humour:

'I wouldn't be seen dead in that outfit!' (Referring to clothes to be buried in.)

'I will die if you say that about me [at the funeral]!'

'I want to look my best when I am dead!'

'Pack my fags just in case…!'

'If you fight like this while I am dying I hate to think what you will do when I am dead!' (A mother to her adult children.)

'Can't you let a man die in peace?' said he when asked to have a wash.

'I am going to my Last Supper,' said a woman who was being taken to a restaurant by her family.

'If I'm going to die I don't want healthy food – buy me a pizza!'

Is palliative care a form of euthanasia?

There is confusion in the minds of many people as to whether palliative care is just another form of euthanasia. The Oxford Dictionary defines euthanasia as 'a gentle and easy death' whereas The Macquarie Dictionary definition is the 'putting of a person to death painlessly'. Both are too vague to be of any help and so I offer the following alternative: Euthanasia is the act of painlessly terminating the life and suffering of another person who is dying from an incurable illness or suffering intolerable pain.

So, what is it about palliative care that has some people accusing it of being nothing less than euthanasia? Consider the following scenario: a 50-year-old woman with advanced cancer of the lung is unconscious and unable to take anything by mouth. She has required morphine in the past to control her pain. As she is now unable to swallow, morphine is given by injection under the skin to ensure she remains pain-free, but all other medications are ceased. An intravenous drip has not been set up, but her mouth and lips are kept moist. She is turned regularly and every effort is made to maintain her dignity, but ultimately she develops a chest infection. Given the situation and her previously expressed wish that she be allowed to die, antibiotics are not given and she dies several days later.

There are several issues in this scenario that could lead some people to ask, is this 'passive' euthanasia? Let's start by saying something about the use of the descriptors 'active' and 'passive' in relation to euthanasia. 'Active' implies a deliberate action and, in the context of euthanasia, this usually involves the administration of a chemical with the expressed purpose of ending a person's life quickly and peacefully – this was the practice followed when euthanasia was legal in the Northern Territory. 'Passive' euthanasia on the other hand is mistakenly used to describe death that comes about because of the failure to implement an action (in this case, setting up an intravenous drip or giving antibiotics) or as a side effect of treatment (in this case, morphine).

The justification for not administering fluids or antibiotics in situations similar to that described is simple. The person is dying and these forms of treatment are not only futile, but are also contrary to the expressed wishes of the patient. The same logic may also apply to the non-use of artificial feeding or the cessation of kidney dialysis or withdrawal of previously beneficial treatment such as heart medication. In all cases the intention is not to end life but to avoid or withdraw treatment that, given the circumstances, is futile. None of these actions meet the definition of euthanasia. Instead, they each represent a form of humane care that is ethically, legally and morally correct in the context of dying. It is good palliative care.

Apart from it being ethically, morally and legally not permissible, active euthanasia, or the deliberate shortening of another person's life (by another), is contrary to the philosophy of palliative care and all that it stands for. It has no place whatsoever in palliative care.

Assisted suicide and assisted dying

Assisted suicide (AS) and assisted dying (AD) are different names used to describe the same action (I prefer AD because it avoids the emotional overtones associated with the word 'suicide'). The typical AD scenario is as follows. A person suffering from a terminal illness and/or intractable pain intentionally kills him/herself, but only with the indirect help of another. The 'other' person may be a doctor who supplies the person with drugs knowing they will be used to end their life. It may also be a friend who seeks out and supplies the person with a cache of lethal drugs (most commonly phenobarbitone). AD is therefore different to euthanasia in that the patient him/herself ends their life even though the means for this has been made available by some other person. As mentioned above euthanasia is when someone other than the patient ends the patient's life as painlessly and quickly as possible. So with AD it is the patient who performs the lethal act but with euthanasia it is someone else, usually a doctor.

At the present time there are only three countries (Belgium, the Netherlands and Switzerland) and three American states (Oregon, Washington and Montana) that have legalised physician-assisted suicide or AD.

A person's right to die was, if you will excuse the pun, brought to life in Australia when, in August 2009, the West Australia Supreme Court handed down a landmark ruling which effectively gave a quadriplegic man the means to die by permitting him to starve to death. Because he depended on others to feed him, this meant the nursing home responsible for his care would not be subject to legal proceedings if they abided by his wishes to starve. While this was a one-off ruling it has certainly reopened the debate on the right to die and has put palliative care in the spotlight once again.

The vast majority of palliative care providers (myself included) do not support AD as it is defined above. They do, however, respect the rights of the terminally ill to refuse treatment, particularly treatment that prolongs dying. I, personally, have no qualms about a terminally ill person not eating, and am comfortable with this stance because it is the disease and not the lack of food that always results in death (see Chapter 5). I have already talked about the use of morphine and other drugs when someone is dying, but because it is so important, let me reiterate. They are used for the expressed purpose of relieving suffering and not to cause death, even though death may occur a little earlier because of their use. This is good palliative care and humane treatment and differs from euthanasia and AD in that they are not used for the expressed purpose of causing death.

Morphine and other morphine-like drugs (opioids) and the question of euthanasia

As far as morphine is concerned, there is now indisputable evidence that people who require pain relief during their illness will experience pain if that medication is ceased. Morphine, given in appropriate doses and for the right reason, will not kill anyone, and failure to administer it when someone is in pain is not only bad practice, it is also unethical and denies a person the very basic human right of pain relief.

Pain is a common complication of chronic illness, not only of cancer and other life-limiting illnesses but also of dementia. Morphine and other morphine-like drugs (opioids) are currently the most effective agents available to counter severe pain. The regular administration of opioids prevents pain but does not eliminate the source of pain. If cancer (or another life-limiting illness) is still present – as it clearly is in those who are dying – pain will resurface if the medication is ceased. Even when unconscious, a person can still perceive pain (see Chapter 6, 'States of consciousness') and appropriate medication must be continued if pain is to be avoided. In the circumstances, injection is the only option available. The dose given should be the smallest amount required to control the pain, but in some cases this may, by necessity, be relatively large.

If a person dies immediately after an injection of morphine, it is not unusual for those present at the time to believe death resulted from the injection. Let me assure you here and now, this is not the case. Death is caused by the underlying disease and the fact it occurred close to the time of the injection is purely coincidental. There is now considerable research to show that morphine given to people who are dying relieves pain and contributes to a peaceful state, but does not cause death. Some research I carried out several years ago showed that people receiving morphine were more peaceful around the time of death than those who were not receiving it.

When given to relieve pain, the risk of respiratory depression secondary to opioids is virtually non-existent as pain itself is a respiratory stimulant and counteracts the problem. In contrast, morphine, heroin or any opioid used for recreational purposes and administered directly into a vein greatly increases the risk of respiratory depression and death. This danger lays not so much with the drug itself but the method of administration and the dose given. Opioids are rarely administered intravenously in the palliative care situation. If it cannot be swallowed it is given by injection under the skin (subcutaneous). The rate of absorption by this route is much too slow to cause serious respiratory depression (see Chapter 3, 'Living with pain').

Many of my patients have required extremely large doses of an opioid to control their pain. Despite the large dose these individuals were not only pain-free, they were also alert and enjoyed a better quality of life. In some instances, drowsiness can be a problem. From my experience this often lessens with continued use of the opioid. If it does not improve, the dose can be reduced. If pain does not permit a dose reduction, an alternative opioid can be tried.

Other medications, particularly sedatives, are sometimes linked with passive euthanasia. As with opioids, sedation is only administered after informed consent is obtained from the patient and/or the family, and then, the dose given is the smallest amount needed to relieve the distress. If these criteria are met and the doctor's intention is to relieve suffering, the use of morphine or any other drug when someone is dying is good palliative care and *not* euthanasia.

Cessation of non-essential medication and euthanasia

Swallowing becomes increasingly difficult when someone is dying and medications, particularly if in large numbers, can become burdensome. In this situation, only those medications required for pain relief or comfort are continued (and administered by injection under the skin), and all other forms of treatment are ceased. This may include tablets for heart trouble, blood pressure or blood clots. Their withdrawal lessens the burden for the dying person and does not significantly influence the time of death. In my experience, almost every sick or dying person expressed relief when the number of pills they were expected to swallow was reduced.

Intravenous/subcutaneous fluids and euthanasia

The use of intravenous or subcutaneous fluids is covered in more detail in Chapter 5, 'Day-to-day care'. Intravenous or subcutaneous fluids do not make a dying person feel better (e.g. relieve thirst) and may introduce new and unwanted problems. Fluids may or may not prolong life, and if they do, it is only by a matter of days. Whether this justifies their use is not a medical decision but a question of choice for the person concerned and the family. Suffice to say here, people do not die from dehydration. They die from the disease that made it difficult or impossible for them to drink.

Withholding antibiotics and euthanasia

I am frequently asked, why do people with cancer die? This is not as strange as it sounds. Is it the cancer, does their heart just give up or is there some other reason? It can be any or all of these, but what usually tips the balance is an underlying infection, p articularly a chest infection. Pneumonia is a very common amongst the sick and the elderly, particularly if the person is unconscious or debilitated from the effects of a prolonged illness. Sir William Osler, a great physician at the turn of the last century described pneumonia as 'the old man's [person's] friend' for it then (and now) guaranteed a quick and painless release for the dying.

One hundred years ago the decision to treat or not treat pneumonia was not a big deal for there were no such things as antibiotics, ventilators and intensive care units. The situation is much more complex today and the decision to treat is an ethical matter as much as a medical decision. The closer someone is to death the easier it is to accept pneumonia as 'a friend'. Not so at other times. Then the decision for or against treatment is made by the patient or family (depending on circumstances) and only after they have received all the information required to make an informed judgement. What it really comes down to is whether treatment will improve a person's quality of life or simply prolong their dying.

Weighing up the evidence

Allowing people to die with as much comfort and dignity as possible is one of the major goals of palliative care. This inevitably involves the administration of medication to eliminate pain (and other symptoms), and the withholding or withdrawal of any treatment that is considered futile. All decisions regarding treatment are based on the dying person's known or stated wishes. If that is not possible the immediate family make a surrogate decision on behalf of their dying relative.

Palliative care offers a holistic and humane way of caring for someone who is dying. It neither hastens nor delays death and seeks only to ease the pain while the process of dying follows its natural course. The quality of a person's life, the dignity of their dying and a respect for their legitimate choices are the major factors that guide the delivery of care. Palliative care, euthanasia and assisted dying all seek to ensure a painless death for those who are dying, but this is all they have in common. The way each achieves this goal is vastly different. Only with palliative care does death occur naturally.

How does palliative care respond to a dying person's request for euthanasia or assisted dying?

A request for euthanasia by a dying person is not only a request for their life to be terminated but also a call for help. Ilora Finlay, a well respected palliative care physician, says that behind most requests for euthanasia is an almost unshakable fear of the future being worse than the present. To see euthanasia then as a problem that must be solved overlooks the need for that person to talk about the overwhelming emotions that lie behind this thinly disguised cry for help. A request for euthanasia flags deep-seated issues that make death appear more acceptable and less frightening than life itself. These issues include fear of suffering, loss of dignity, a sense of hopelessness, uncertainty about the future and the meaningless of their life. In some cases the request arises because the dying person is ready to die but mistakenly believes treatment is prolonging their life. Some feel they have become a burden to their family, particularly to those responsible for their day-to-day care. For these and other reasons they see a quick and painless death as the best solution to the problem.

Because of the many possible scenarios that underlie a request for euthanasia, the best response is to allow the person to tell their story, to express their fears and concerns, and to ensure they are heard. For many, the plea is not that they be killed but that they are allowed to die and that nothing out of the ordinary is done to prolong their life – in other words they seek good palliative care. For a small number, the desire for euthanasia is real, but the opportunity to talk is, often all that is needed.

There are, however a few who persist in their request and if it is not met, or if their despair goes unheard, they may attempt suicide or seek outside help to end their life. The desperation and sense of abandonment these individuals must feel is unimaginable. I have cared for several people who did not want to go on living but were equally afraid of death. Never have I felt so helpless. Their despair was seemingly insoluble and nothing their family or I did was of any help. Two of these people died in unfortunate circumstances but several others improved once I started to listen and stopped trying to solve their problem. To paraphrase Teilhard de Chardin, the difficulty for them was not how to solve the problem but how to express it.

The carer's role in this situation is very difficult. Your thoughts and feelings may be so entangled it is often hard to see a way through. This is a time when you will benefit from talking to a friend or a counsellor, not about solutions but about the way you feel. Your load becomes a little bit lighter if you can share it with someone you trust.

Chapter 3

Living with pain

Unless we look the beast in the eye
we will find that it returns
to hold us hostage

DESMOND TUTU
No future without forgiveness

Chapter 3

Living with pain

When someone first receives a diagnosis of a life-threatening illness their whole world is turned upside down and they are overwhelmed by painful thoughts and emotions. In the midst of this chaos two things commonly stand out – a dread of what the future holds, and the thought of dying in pain. This is particularly true if the diagnosis is cancer. The association between cancer, death and pain is deeply entrenched in many of us, and the mere mention of the word 'cancer' becomes a death sentence rather than a diagnosis. The fear cancer invokes is at times a bigger problem than the disease itself, creating enormous personal and family grief and a future that at best remains uncertain. Although pain is not so prominent in other life-threatening illnesses, fear of the unknown and fear of death are just as real and damaging as they are with cancer.

In this chapter I will talk more about cancer pain and its treatment, and explore the ramifications of pain beyond the physical domain. I hope to dispel many of the myths and misconceptions that not only compromise care, but also result in unnecessary pain and hardship. I will conclude by exploring what I call the pain of dying, and how this impacts on the life of the carer and the 'cared for'. The following story illustrates the complexity of pain and how it can be influenced by a person's life experience as well as by their illness.

Lou was an elderly man with a long and complicated medical history. He was found to have cancer of the prostate that had, at diagnosis, already spread to his bones, causing moderately severe pain. As his health deteriorated he went from one specialist to another and despite first-rate medical attention and good pain relief he became very depressed. It seemed the cancer was robbing him of more than his health. His inability to do the things he loved and his increasing dependence on others led him to believe he was a nuisance, a burden, and better dead than alive. Lou was more afraid of life than death and he now longed to die. This greatly disturbed his family, who were unsure how to resolve the dilemma. Lou often sat alone in his workshop. On one occasion his son wandered in and asked what was troubling him. He caught him at a vulnerable time – Lou was more open than usual and, as was his habit, he resorted to allegory to explain his dilemma...

There was once a sick, elderly man who lived with his only son. One day he said to the son, 'I want you to take me to a place where I can die.' The son knew he was ill but could not understand why he wanted to leave home. The father gave no explanation and persisted with his request. Ultimately, the son gave in, not because he wanted him to leave but because he wanted to see what lay behind his unusual plea. Because he was so weak, the father begged his son to carry him. After several hours they reached the outskirts of town. When they came to a desolate spot the old man asked that he be left there and told his son to return home. The son was alarmed and insisted they both return home. The old man said, 'You must do as I say, as this is where I carried my father and left him to die.'

A dialogue between father and son followed and during this Lou was able to look his beast in the eye. Lou carried an enormous guilt over his own father's death some fifty years earlier and was able to express this through the allegory. Following this disclosure Lou's depression lifted and he was relieved of a burden he had carried all these years. He died shortly after.

The message contained within this story is so powerful there is no need to elaborate. What is important is that some of the most troublesome, yet most overlooked, pains are those that have a non-physical basis. The unveiling of these pains can be as rewarding as the relief of any physical discomfort. Lou broke the shell that had enclosed fifty years of grief and, while the process was painful, the result was liberating. This has had a great impact on my life for Lou was my father and I listened to his story and shared his grief and ultimate healing.

It is surprising how many people carry painful memories that have been neatly locked away in their subconscious in order for them to survive (psychologically speaking). No matter what the memory or how deep it is, it commonly comes to the surface when that person confronts their own mortality. It will then manifest in any number of ways, but often as depression, despair, extreme fear or anxiety. A medical approach will, as with Lou, always fall short, for what is needed is for the person to revisit their past. The source of their angst may be anything from the experience of a concentration camp, incarceration, torture, abuse or abandonment, but it could also be something relatively minor that falls under the category of 'unfinished business'.

The benefits that come from understanding pain (or suffering) are found in the words of the Dutch philosopher Spinoza, who said, 'Emotion, which is suffering, ceases to be suffering as soon as we form a clear and precise picture of it'. Many times in this book I speak of the journey people make as they confront their own death and how necessary this may be to their own healing. Lou's healing came not only from him forming a clear and precise picture of his suffering but also from sharing it with someone else. And so it is with all forms of healing. You, as family and friends, and we in the health care profession, need to be on the alert for signposts that indicate suffering. Marie De Hennezel in her book *Intimate Death* sums this up beautifully: 'There is a need to give shape to one's life and to show this shape, which gives it its meaning, to someone else. Once the telling of it has been accomplished the person seems to be able to let go and die'.

Pain: what is it?

Pain has been described as an unpleasant sensory and emotional experience that results from some form of damage or injury to the body. In other words, it hurts (sensory experience) and because it hurts we may cry, call out in anger or, in cases of chronic pain such as with cancer, become depressed (emotional experience). This emotional component is much greater in those with chronic pain, particularly if the cause of the pain also threatens that person's life.

The overall experience of pain (sensory plus emotional) is not the same for everyone, even though the source and intensity of the painful stimulus may be similar. Whether we show pain and the way it is expressed depends on many things other than the degree of physical discomfort. These include personal and cultural factors, learnt experiences and the circumstances surrounding the pain. Some will endure considerable pain before they complain while others will exhibit pain behaviour (e.g. cry) simply because they anticipate pain – a child about to receive an injection is a good example of the latter.

When someone complains of pain, particularly in the context of cancer, it is helpful to see their pain as the tip of an iceberg. The amount of pain 'showing' depends not only on the underlying disease (physical), but also on other factors (Figure 3.1). As the other elements operate below the surface they are easily overlooked, but are nonetheless important in the overall experience and treatment of pain. The 'iceberg' model helps us to see pain in its entirety, and to appreciate the importance of holistic care.

If the social, emotional and spiritual needs of the person are ignored or if the environment worsens (e.g. becomes noisier), pain may seem worse even though the physical component may be unchanged. Pain can worsen with the progression of disease but it is important to realise that the overall experience of pain results not just from illness but from a complex interaction of the physical, emotional, social and spiritual state of a person.

As we come to appreciate the nature of pain, the word itself seems perfunctory for it fails to convey its complexity. Some have described pain as either physical (when it arises from a physical cause) or spiritual (when it has a social, emotional or spiritual basis). This is misleading, as it is uncommon for either pain to exist in a pure form. They nearly always coexist, particularly with chronic pain. The word 'suffering' incorporates both the physical and the psycho-spiritual dimensions of pain and the rawness of the word conveys the undeniable message that we are dealing with a complex human experience. 'Suffering' rather than 'pain' is the more appropriate term to use when describing a chronic pain situation.

The following sections focus on some of the physical aspects of pain, but we should not forget how important the non-physical dimensions are in the expression of pain and suffering.

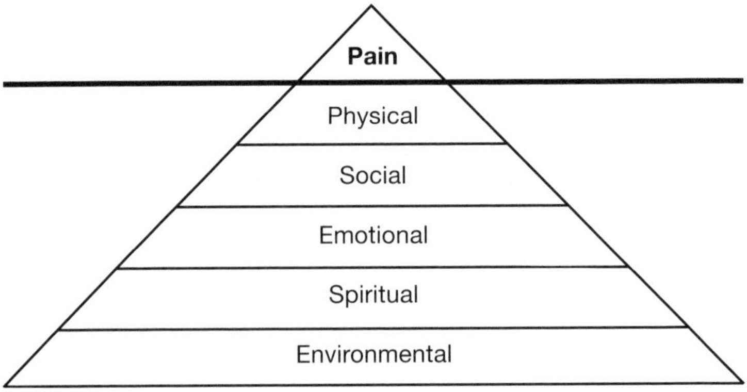

FIGURE 3.1 The 'iceberg' model of pain, showing pain as the tip of an iceberg. How much pain is expressed depends on the presence and magnitude of the factors beneath the surface.

How does cancer cause pain?

Cancer is an abnormal growth of cells within the body. This growth generally starts in one organ and the cancer derives its name from that organ – for example, cancer of the lung means the cancer originated in the lung. Cancers grow and spread locally to lymph glands and later to distant organs such as the liver, bones and the brain. As the cancer grows it ultimately compresses or invades surrounding structures, resulting in pain or a worsening of pain. The amount of pain experienced depends on the degree of pressure and the structures that are affected. It is usually worse if bones or nerves are involved. How much the person complains of pain is, of course, another matter.

When cancer spreads from its original site to other organs (e.g. lung cancer that spreads to bone or the liver), the cancer in these new sites is still lung cancer. It is not bone cancer or liver cancer. Secondary spread, in medical parlance, is most commonly referred to as a *metastasis* if solitary or *metastases* if multiple. In our example, the correct medical terminology would be cancer of the lung with bone and liver metastases.

Cancer pain is typically chronic and unremitting, and persists for as long as the cancer is present. In the vast majority of cases the pain responds to conventional pain-relieving medication (analgesics). The pain may worsen over time but is usually controlled with adjustments in the dose of analgesics. A sudden worsening may indicate disease progression or a related or unrelated complication. What is important is that the doctor looks for an explanation for the sudden worsening and does not increase the dose of analgesics mindlessly. This applies equally to pain resulting from any chronic or potentially life-threatening illness.

Determining the cause of pain

Before deciding on the most appropriate treatment your doctor will always exclude pain from other sources and will not automatically assume it is due to cancer or some other known disease. In the case of cancer, not all pains are due to the cancer and to assume otherwise may result in inappropriate treatment and potentially serious consequences. For example, a blood clot in the lung not only requires treatment to ease the pain but also specific medication to prevent further clots. The examples of David and Ashley illustrate the importance of determining the exact cause of pain.

David had been in the palliative care ward for several weeks. He had cancer of the lung that had spread to his bones, resulting in considerable pain. The pain slowly improved with analgesics, and although not completely pain-free he was able to move around the ward with the minimum of support. One morning he woke with a new and troublesome pain in the right hip. Knowing the cancer had spread to David's bones, the doctor assumed this was the cause of the new pain and ordered an injection of morphine. Before the injection was given the nurse asked the doctor to return to David's bedside and check on something she had noticed. In the bed was a biro top that David had obviously been lying on for some time. This had not only left its mark on his skin but was also responsible for the pain. Once the pen top had been removed and David repositioned, the pain quickly settled.

Ashley had melanoma that had spread throughout his body. One weekend he developed pain in the lower part of his abdomen. Despite an injection of morphine the pain worsened and continued despite two further injections. He was admitted to the local palliative care ward where he was found to have an enlarged bladder. As he was unable to pass urine, a catheter was inserted and a large volume of urine drained, with immediate relief of the pain.

In both examples the pain resolved rapidly once the cause had been determined and appropriate action taken. Neither required an increase in analgesics, and in Ashley's case the inappropriate use of morphine resulted in unnecessary delay and suffering. Anything other than minor aches and pains need to be assessed thoroughly before a decision about treatment can be made.

The best assessment involves listening to a person's description of pain and then making a physical examination, taking particular note of body language. It is hard to let others know how much pain we are experiencing. Restlessness, grimaces and an unusual posture may say more about a person's pain than the words used to describe it. Similarly, pain that interferes with sleep or limits activity is strong indirect evidence of severe pain. The opposite also applies. Someone who appears comfortable and smiles as they tell me about their pain makes me think outside the square and to evaluate the pain very carefully. Tests may be helpful, particularly if there is some uncertainty as to the cause of the pain, but they should never be a substitute for listening and looking.

How common is pain at the end of life?

Contrary to popular belief, pain is not a universal accompaniment of cancer. Approximately 80 per cent will experience pain at some stage of their illness. Clearly this means 20 per cent do not. Although pain is not a feature of other life-threatening illnesses, it can occur. When it does it is usually milder than cancer pain and settles with relatively small does of analgesics. Having said that, I have cared for many people with heart conditions, strokes or AIDS who had severe pain and required large doses of morphine.

Of those that get pain, the majority can expect good to excellent pain relief from conventional analgesics. A certain proportion, possibly 10 per cent, have pain that is more difficult to eradicate and requires a larger doses of analgesics or a combination of medications to achieve relief. A much smaller number – usually people with cancer – have intractable pain that does not respond or responds poorly to currently available treatment.

Unrelieved pain can have devastating effects on an individual, leading in some instances to a sense of hopelessness and despair. Ultimately, this may prove to be as destructive as the pain itself. Whatever the cause or the severity we must always interpret pain carefully and respond immediately and appropriately.

Guidelines for the treatment of cancer pain

If an analgesic is required to relieve pain, the earlier it is started the better. Pain is easier to control and the required dose is smaller when treatment is not delayed. People do not need to suffer nor do they have to 'earn' their pain relief. If you know or even suspect your relative/friend has pain, encourage them to see a doctor – they may be reluctant to do so for one or more of these reasons:

- fear of what may be causing the pain
- fear that pain signifies impending death
- fear of commencing analgesics
- wishful thinking (hoping the pain will go away)
- denial (believing the pain is due to something else)
- stoicism (accepting that the pain is due to cancer but unwilling to have pain relief).

Treatment for pain is given regularly (to prevent pain), not just when pain is present. The dose required over a 24-hour period is generally less and the pain better controlled if analgesics are given in this way. To take analgesics when there is no pain is a hard concept to grasp but the logic is simple. Analgesics suppress pain but do not eliminate the source of the pain. So, even if an analgesic succeeds in relieving pain, the pain will return once the analgesic has washed out of the system. Depending on the analgesic, this 'washout' time may be as short as four hours or as long as one week. The aim is to repeat the analgesic before the previous dose loses its effect. You will receive clear directions on how this is done, and it is advisable to get all instructions in writing.

Your doctor will always start with a relatively small dose of an analgesic. This minimises side effects but also ensures your relative will get the smallest dose that does the job. The dose will be increased slowly over a matter of days until pain relief is achieved. Do not be alarmed if the pain does not settle immediately. It often takes several days to a week before good pain control is secured. If pain is severe, the doctor may start with a slightly higher dose and escalate the dose more rapidly to achieve the desired pain control.

Most analgesics have unwanted side effects. The doctor will go through these and recommend how best to prevent them. Constipation is the most troublesome and occurs with most of the stronger analgesics. More is said about side effects later in the chapter.

You will be given instructions about how to treat any unexpected exacerbation of pain. Such pain is called *breakthrough pain* because it has broken through the analgesic barrier. The extra medication required to control this pain is called 'breakthrough medication' or simply 'a breakthrough'. Approximately two breakthrough doses are permitted in a 24-hour period. If more are required the doctor should be informed as the medication and the situation may need to be reviewed. The section 'Analgesics and pain control' that follows contains more information on breakthrough pain and its treatment. Read it carefully to ensure you have the necessary medication and information.

Call your doctor or palliative care nurse if there is a sudden worsening or unexpected change in the pain. Whether you do this immediately or later will depend on the severity of the pain and the time of day or night. Always err on the side of calling if you are unsure, particularly if pain is severe and has not responded to the recommended breakthrough medication.

Radiotherapy and pain control

Radiotherapy utilises high energy X-rays to target the cancer with a view to relieving symptoms (palliative radiotherapy) or to produce a cure (curative radiotherapy). Unfortunately, there are few situations where radiotherapy is curative and more often than not it is used to ease the pain or other distressing symptoms associated with cancer. It does this by shrinking the cancer and thereby relieving pressure on surrounding structures. It is most effective and most frequently used to ease pain from cancer deposits within the bone. It is also used to shrink cancer in and around vital areas, such as the brain, spinal cord, pelvis and lung.

Because the benefits of radiotherapy often appear several weeks after completion, analgesics are continued during this time, but may be reduced if and when the treatment has the desired effect. Rarely can the analgesics be ceased altogether.

Radiotherapy may be delivered over one or more sessions. The overall health of the person and the site of pain are two of many factors that determine which is preferable. Radiotherapy delivered in one session is obviously more convenient for someone in pain and gives quicker results. Some areas of the body are highly sensitive to radiotherapy and are not suited to this single treatment. Treatment to these sites must be given over several days or weeks to avoid damage to the surrounding normal tissues. The radiotherapy doctor can advise you further on this matter.

Side effects depend on the amount of radiotherapy given and the site that is irradiated. Some areas are much more susceptible to the effects of radiotherapy, for example the brain, lung, liver, oesophagus and mouth. Nausea is perhaps the most common side effect, but is often preventable if appropriate prophylactic medication is given. Redness of the skin and inflammation of mucosal surfaces (mouth, oesophagus) may also occur. Alopecia is inevitable when radiotherapy is directed to the head or brain. The radiotherapy department will always speak to you about the treatment and its side effects. Information booklets are also available from the radiotherapy department.

Analgesics and pain control

If pain is troublesome or persistent, pain-relieving medication (analgesics) will almost certainly be prescribed by the doctor. As much as everyone wants relief from pain, the introduction of analgesics often raises questions and concerns that need to be addressed. These concerns are greatest if morphine is the recommended medication, particularly if this is the first time the dreaded 'M' word has been used. Most people associate its use with impending death or believe it may hasten death or lead to addiction. These are just some of the many myths and misconceptions that are addressed later in this chapter.

The number and range of analgesics has increased dramatically in recent years. Morphine remains the gold standard against which others are measured, but patient fears about its use and the emergence of equally effective analgesics have seen a change in the prescribing habits of GPs and specialists.

Commonly used analgesics

- **Paracetamol**, known commercially as Panadol®, is frequently used in the palliative care situation to relieve minor pains. Although a weak analgesic, paracetamol can potentiate the effect of stronger analgesics such as morphine and is often used in combination with it (or other strong analgesics). Paracetamol alone is particularly good for pleurisy and, like aspirin, can lower the temperature in someone who has a fever. It comes as a tablet, capsule or in liquid form. Some people find the tablets hard to swallow, and with a recommended dose of six to twelve tablets a day this may be more than a sick person can tolerate. Paracetamol, even in this dose, is safe except for those with severe liver disease
- **Aspirin.** Aspirin is as good an analgesic as paracetamol, but is not often used in palliative care because it also 'thins the blood'. This

increases the risk of bleeding in someone with a serious illness, particularly leukaemia. This blood-thinning property is used to advantage in those with heart or circulation problems, but aspirin is potentially risky and rarely used as an analgesic in the palliative care situation. Its use is contraindicated in young children.

- **Panadeine Forte®.** This combination of paracetamol and codeine is more potent than paracetamol alone but significantly weaker than morphine and other opioids such as oxycodone and fentanyl. Panadeine Forte® is extremely constipating and this side effect limits its usefulness.
- **Tramadol** is as potent as Panadeine Forte® but has the advantage of being less constipating. It is available as a short-acting capsule and long-acting tablet or as an injection. Tramadol is occasionally used for mild to moderate pain. It is often prescribed by general practitioners who are looking for an analgesic more potent than paracetamol but weaker than morphine.
- **Non-steroidal anti-inflammatory agents** are frequently prescribed for the treatment of painful arthritis, but are also used in the palliative care situation for bone pain – usually in combination with other analgesics. They come in tablet and capsule form, and also an injection. Non-steroidal anti-inflammatory drugs have several side effects and should be avoided if someone has a bleeding tendency or history of high blood pressure, kidney disease or stomach/duodenal ulcers. Care should also be taken if they are used in combination with drugs commonly prescribed for high blood pressure or ankle swelling.
- **Fentanyl** is one of the newer long-acting analgesics. It is widely used in palliative care and for people who have chronic pain. It has several attributes that make it attractive to patients and to the doctors that prescribe it. Fentanyl is absorbed through the skin so, rather than having to swallow tablets, a patch is applied to the upper arm or trunk and replaced every 72 hours. Fentanyl is

less constipating and less sedating than other strong analgesics, and can be used when someone is unable to swallow. It comes in several strengths and while useful for mild to severe pain it is not recommended when pain is unstable.

When applying the patch it is important to ensure the full circumference adheres well to the skin. If the seal is incomplete, the patch may be less effective or may lose potency well before the 72 hours. In some situations, the patch may not give a full 72 hours pain relief even when the seal is perfect. For this reason you should speak to the doctor or nurse if pain is worse during the last 24 hours of the patch's application.

The rate at which the drug is absorbed increases if the patch is exposed to the sun or receives the full force of a hot shower. The same effect is noted in hot climates – in the Northern Territory, for example, it is not uncommon for patches to be changed every 24 to 48 hours. There are also situations where the amount of drug absorbed through the skin may be less than expected. This occurs when someone has lost a lot of weight or if their circulation is very poor. If your loved one is prescribed fentanyl patches, discuss these important practical issues with your doctor or community nurse. Fentanyl also comes as a quick-acting lozenge (lollypop) that can be used for sudden or breakthrough pain. It is available on the Pharmaceutical Benefit Scheme but supply is limited.

- **Norspan®** is similar to fentanyl in that it comes as a patch, but differs in that it has a longer duration of action (one week). It, too, comes in several strengths, making it a weak-moderate strength analgesic. Its profile makes it particularly useful for the aged population and for someone who requires something more than paracetamol, but has not quite reached the stage of requiring morphine or its equivalent. Norspan® is occasionally used in combination with other analgesics. All the practical points concerning fentanyl patches also apply to Norspan®.

- **Hydromorphone** is a very potent analgesic. It is relatively new to Australia, but has been available and used in the USA for quite some time. Hydromorphone comes as a liquid (Dilaudud®), long-acting tablets (Jurnista®) and an injection. Initially it was reserved for people unable to tolerate morphine or oxycodone, but because of its effectiveness and safety, it is now commonly prescribed first up.
- **Methadone.** Once rarely used in the palliative care situation it is now commonly prescribed for specific situations. Methadone has a complex metabolism and its tolerance and dosage varies from one individual to another. This has, to date, limited its use, but as palliative care doctors become more familiar with its idiosyncrasies it will be prescribed more often, particularly for 'nerve' pain or for those unable to tolerate other analgesics.
- **Heroin.** Some people mistakenly believe heroin is a better analgesic than morphine and should be available for those with severe pain. Heroin is simply two morphine molecules joined together (diamorphine) and once in the body it is metabolised into morphine. Heroin is therefore morphine by another name and is equivalent to morphine in its potency. It is used in the United Kingdom, not because it is any better than morphine, but because it is more soluble. This means the volume of heroin required for injection is smaller than that for an equivalent dose of morphine. Heroin is not available for medical use within Australia.
- **Pethidine** is a good analgesic when pain is acute, as with trauma or immediately after surgery. It is not recommended nor should it be used when pain relief is required over a prolonged period of time as is the case with cancer or chronic pain. Pethidine has a brief duration of action and potentially toxic breakdown products that can accumulate with continuous use. For these reasons it is rarely if ever used in palliative care.
- **Marijuana** (cannabis). While there is nothing more than anecdotal evidence to suggest that marijuana helps cancer or non-cancer pain,

research continues to probe this somewhat controversial subject. Marijuana cannot be legally prescribed in Australia. Possession of a small amount for personal use has been decriminalised in the ACT, NT, SA and WA, but its possession and use still remains a criminal offence in the remaining states (Google *NDARC fact sheet* and search for *cannabis and the law*). Most people who use marijuana for pain relief rarely use it as the sole analgesic agent. It is usually an unconventional addition to other conventional analgesics. While it should never be first-line treatment, I can understand why people with a painful or life-threatening illness may wish to try it.

- **Oxycodone** is now the most commonly prescribed analgesic for the relief of all types of pain. It is as potent as morphine, and although its side effect profile is similar, it has little of the stigma associated with morphine. Oxycodone is available as a short-acting tablet (Endone®), capsule or liquid (Oxynorm®) and as a longer-acting tablet (Oxycontin®). A wide range of strengths allows your doctor to fine tune the dose of oxycodone by simply changing the strength of the preparation rather than increasing the number of tablets. Unlike the long-acting form of morphine, Oxycontin® has a biphasic action, meaning its effect is noticeable within 20 minutes of swallowing and lasts for a full 12 hours (occasionally 8 hours). As with long-acting morphine, Oxycontin® tablets should be swallowed whole and not chewed or crushed. An injectable form of oxycodone, for those who cannot swallow, is available, but cost limits its use.
- **Morphine** is one of the oldest and most effective analgesics and is used, not only for cancer pain, but also for chronic non-malignant pain that does not respond to simpler analgesics. Like oxycodone, morphine is available in the short-acting (liquid Ordine®) and long-acting forms (MS Contin® or Kapanol®), and also as an injection. All the formulations come in different strengths and so a dose increase simply means a stronger strength tablet or liquid rather than a greater number of tablets or increased volume of liquid. When

prescribing morphine, the doctor will often start with Ordine®. Although Ordine® has to be taken every 4 hours the inconvenience of frequent dosing is made up for by quicker and better pain control. Because of its rapid onset of action (20 minutes after swallowing), Ordine® is also prescribed routinely for breakthrough pain.

Ordine® has a bitter taste but this can be largely overcome by mixing it with juice or other drinks, but not alcohol. Short-acting morphine is also available in the more convenient tablet form, Sevredol® and Anamorph®, and these may, at times, be used as a substitute for Ordine®. Long-acting morphine is usually substituted for the short-acting form once pain has been controlled. Unlike Ordine® or its tablet equivalent, these preparations take several hours to reach their maximum effect. This slow onset of action renders them unsuitable for breakthrough pain. Long-acting tablets and capsules must be swallowed whole and not chewed. If someone has difficulty swallowing, a long-acting morphine suspension is available, or alternatively the contents of the morphine capsule can be sprinkled onto ice cream or yoghurt and then swallowed. Morphine injections are used if a person is unable to swallow or if they are vomiting. For more information on morphine injections, speak to one of the doctors or nurses involved in your relative's care. Like most analgesics, morphine is extremely constipating and almost all patients will require daily laxatives to prevent this complication.

Morphine myths

One fears only what one does not understand.

ANTON CHEKHOV

Patients and their families usually have mixed feelings when pain-relieving medication is suggested or prescribed for the first time. The relief of knowing that something can be done to ease pain is tempered by the realisation that he/she has now entered another phase of the illness, and that their life may be dominated by pain and the medication required to combat it. There may also be a fear of addiction or of becoming excessively sedated or that the introduction of this type of medication heralds the beginning of the end. Much of this fear, certainly in relation to morphine, is based on myth, hearsay and misunderstanding. For some the mere mention of the 'M' word causes as much alarm as does the word cancer. The newer analgesics have not been around long enough to become part of this folklore, and are generally better accepted by patients and their relatives.

Misconceptions can sometimes delay the introduction of necessary treatment and contribute to protracted suffering. Sadly, it is the family rather than the person in pain that has most difficulty in accepting the need for morphine, and not infrequently they baulk at the mere mention of the word. This resistance not only stems from misunderstanding and fear, but may also be part of a family's grief. Whatever the reason, talking usually helps resolve the situation.

The following Question and Answer section might help you to better understand many of the issues you are concerned about, dispel some of the fear, and give you the confidence to use morphine safely and correctly. I will use the word morphine throughout this coming section, but what is said applies equally to any of the strong analgesics. So, if your relative is on oxycodone, fentanyl, hydromorphone or methadone, et cetera, substitute that analgesic whenever you read the word 'morphine'.

Is morphine addictive?

Yes and no. If morphine is administered directly into the vein for a sufficiently long period of time it may result in addiction. Given this way, morphine, like many other drugs, produces an immediate euphoria and it is this that makes it addictive. Morphine is rarely if ever administered into the vein in a palliative care situation. It is nearly always given by mouth as a tablet, capsule or liquid or as an injection under the skin (or as a patch, in the case of fentanyl and Norspan®). Absorption is much too slow by any of these routes to induce euphoria and so the risk of addiction is virtually zero. Caution must be exercised in those who have a recent or past addiction to morphine, heroin or some other drug, but even then morphine, if required for pain relief, can be used safely and effectively.

If morphine is started early in the course of an illness, will it work when it is really needed?

Morphine will continue to work for as long as it is given. If a dose increase is required, this is because the underlying condition has worsened, resulting in more pain. A dose increase is never due to the drug becoming less effective. It is not uncommon for palliative care patients to be on morphine for months or years, and even over this length of time tolerance does not develop.

Does starting morphine now mean the end is near?

Morphine may be recommended at any stage of an illness if symptoms are present that will benefit from its introduction. Its use does not mean death is near, only that a better quality of life is possible. It is true that morphine is commonly used when someone is dying. Many, if not all of these people required morphine well before this time and its continued use ensures their ongoing comfort.

Can morphine be used for symptoms other than pain?

Morphine can ease the distress associated with breathlessness and is, perhaps the best cough suppressant available. For these reasons it may be helpful for those who have advanced heart disease, emphysema or cancer of the lung. The dose required to treat breathlessness and cough is often much smaller than that required for pain, and can sometimes be miniscule. Despite earlier unfounded concerns, its safety and efficacy in heart and lung disease is now confirmed.

Is morphine safe?

As with any drug, the safety of morphine depends on it being prescribed for the right reason and in a dose appropriate to the circumstances. Occasionally someone may have an unexpected response to the drug –

this may be because of a previously unknown allergy or an unexpected sensitivity. As far as morphine is concerned, a true allergy is rare. Sensitivity to morphine is more common that allergy. This often manifests as sleepiness or confusion following relatively small doses of the drug. If this occurs, a dose reduction or cessation of the drug is all that is required. Having said this, morphine is remarkably safe and its benefits, particularly in the palliative care situation, are unquestioned. Reports of morphine killing or being used to kill someone always involve inappropriately large doses, often by injection into a vein, and usually for recreational purposes rather than a medical reason. After more than 40 years medical practice I have not had one instance where morphine has been directly responsible for a person's death.

Is it safe to use morphine for long periods?

Morphine can be used safely and effectively for long periods. Its analgesic effect does not diminish over time. The fact it is recommended and approved by statutory bodies for the treatment of chronic pain associated with non-life-threatening illnesses speaks volumes for its safety.

Is morphine safe when given in large doses?

Those with severe pain usually require a larger than average dose of morphine. This dose will be arrived at over time and a slow escalation generally reduces the likelihood of unacceptable side effects such as drowsiness and confusion. Used carefully and correctly, morphine is absolutely safe, even in these large doses – the biggest worry is the underlying illness that creates the need for a dose increase. Recent research has suggested that with some people requiring large doses of morphine for pain control, the problem may not be the disease but the person's genetic makeup. These people metabolise morphine in such a way as to render it less effective. This discovery may explain a situation that has puzzled me for many years. I was once asked to see a young woman who, despite massive doses of morphine, still complained of severe pain. I was surprised by the dose, (the largest dose of any patient I have ever treated) and the fact she still had pain. The greatest surprise, however, was that she was wide awake, with no signs of morphine overdose.

Can some other analgesic be used in place of morphine?

There are now many alternatives to morphine. Most are similar to morphine in their action, efficacy and side effects and may for a variety of reasons be preferred or substituted for it. Morphine is often recommended because of its proven safety and effectiveness. The newer analgesics have been around long enough to have stood the test of time, and it is now increasingly common for one of them to be offered as a first option or to be substituted for morphine if the latter results in troublesome side effects.

Does a history of morphine allergy mean it cannot be used?

Morphine allergy is extremely rare. Most people with a so-called allergy are told or think they are allergic because they once vomited following an injection, often after an operation. This is not an allergy, but a side effect of the morphine or the operation. It does not preclude further use of morphine, although the concomitant use of an anti-emetic (anti-vomiting agent) would be advisable. In the rare case of true morphine allergy, morphine should be avoided and another analgesic used in its place.

Does morphine cause drowsiness?

As with many other drugs, morphine can result in some drowsiness when it is commenced or when the dose is increased. Any drowsiness generally improves after a few days. If it persists the dose may be reduced, but If that's not possible (because of pain), an alternative analgesic is the only option.

Are there any other side effects of morphine?

The most common side effects of morphine use are dry mouth and constipation. Frequent sips of water are recommended for the former and laxatives are always required to prevent the latter. Nausea and vomiting occur in one third of those taking morphine and can be prevented or controlled by the addition of an anti-emetic. Confusion is less common. It is usually dose related, and can be improved by a dose reduction or, if that is not possible, a change to another analgesic. Muscle twitching is generally of nuisance value for it usually occurs as the person is nodding off to sleep. If severe, the dose of morphine should be reduced, pain permitting. Sweating and itch occur uncommonly, but can be so troublesome as to require a change in analgesics. If the person has cancer, sweating is more likely due to that and not to the morphine.

How will I know if my relative/friend is getting too much morphine?

Signs of morphine toxicity are quite variable, but if any of the following side effects is present it is best to consult your doctor or speak to a community nurse as soon as possible. Side effects commonly associated with morphine toxicity include excessive drowsiness or difficulty in being roused, worsening confusion, unusual behaviour, visual or auditory hallucinations and frequent or violent muscle twitching.

Will side effects occur with other analgesics if they have previously occurred with morphine?

It's possible but the likelihood is less. Because there is no guaranteed way of choosing the best alternative, your doctor may need to try one or more analgesics before the right one is found. It is better to do this than omit analgesics altogether or continue with one that causes troublesome side effects.

What should be done if pain reappears despite regular treatment with morphine?

It is not uncommon for someone on morphine to get occasional or intermittent pain in or around the site of their cancer – this pain is often referred to as breakthrough pain simply because it has broken through the morphine barrier. Because it is a relatively common occurrence your doctor will provide you with what is called 'breakthrough' medication, and advise you on how and when to use it. Immediate relief of pain is the object of the exercise, so breakthrough medication is always the rapid onset, short-acting variety. The longer-acting preparations are not suitable as their onset of action is generally, but not always, too slow to be of value in this situation. The most common analgesics recommended for breakthrough pain are Ordine® (morphine), Endone® and Oxynorm® (oxycodone) and Dilaudid® (hydromorphone).

When breakthrough pain occurs the prescribed breakthrough medication should be taken irrespective of when other analgesics were taken or are due. For example, if someone has moderate-severe pain one hour before the next dose of regular medication, the breakthrough dose should be administered, and the regular analgesic given when it is due. In other words, regular analgesics are never omitted in the face of breakthrough medication.

If pain persists one hour after the breakthrough dose, the dose can be repeated. If the second dose does not relieve the pain, your doctor or community nurse should be contacted.

One to two breakthrough doses over 24 hours is acceptable, but if more is required your doctor will almost certainly review the situation. It helps if you keep a diary of breakthrough medication with the date and times they are administered.

Can a person drive a motor vehicle or continue working while taking morphine?

Driving a car is permitted providing the person is alert and on a stable dose of morphine. With every dose increase, the person should cease driving for a few days until the effect of that increased dose becomes apparent. Much the same applies to work if safety issues are involved. The RTA should be advised about the use of morphine and, subject to the above provisos, problems rarely arise. The driving of buses or trucks is another matter and this needs to be discussed with your doctor.

Can morphine be ceased after it has been commenced?

An easing of the pain does not mean there is no further need for morphine. More often than not the pain is better because of the medication. Stopping treatment will almost certainly result in a rapid and dramatic resurgence of pain. So never stop morphine without discussing it with the person overseeing its use. In the unlikely event of pain improving for reasons other than morphine, the dose will be reduced slowly and carefully, but always under medical supervision.

Why can't morphine be withdrawn abruptly?

If a person has required morphine for some time, stopping it suddenly or reducing the dose rapidly can result in unpleasant symptoms like restlessness, insomnia and sweating. This is a physical withdrawal and does NOT indicate addiction. The same withdrawal symptoms also occur when other commonly prescribed medications are withdrawn suddenly. This also applies to tea, coffee and cigarettes. Addiction is suspected when a person craves for a drug and the craving is associated with antisocial behaviour.

Does this mean morphine has to be taken for the rest of a person's life?

Morphine may need to be taken for the rest of a person's life, not because of the risk of withdrawal, but because the symptom for which it was prescribed will resurface once it is ceased.

Is morphine a dangerous drug?

No more dangerous than any other drug, but as with all drugs, it should be kept in a safe place and certainly out of the reach of children.

How and where should morphine be stored?

Morphine is best stored in a safe, cool place and out of direct sunlight.

Are there any non-drug measures that can be tried to improve pain?

Hot packs may be useful in the treatment of pain but must be used carefully to avoid burns. Massage, therapeutic touch, Reiki, prayer and meditation have been shown to help. Acupuncture and TENS (trans-electrical nerve stimulation) also have a place. TENS is similar to acupuncture in the way it works, but uses low levels of electrical current on the skin in place of needles. All these non-drug measures may help with minor pains but rarely improve the more severe variety. For this reason they are best used in combination with morphine, not as an alternative.

Does morphine relieve any of the angst that may accompany pain?
If the angst is related to pain, pain relief will certainly improve morale and lessen fear – fear that they will have to suffer pain for the rest of their life. If the angst is more deep seated, it will take much more than pain relief to ease this form of suffering. More will be said about this later in the chapter.

Pain that does not respond to morphine

In most instances, pain that responds poorly to morphine has an obvious cause. It may be a result of cancer or any number of illnesses. Patients will often describe this pain as unbearable or beyond belief and their body language will be consistent with the description they give. In some instances words to describe the pain are inadequate and then people may say something like, how long do I have to put up with this, or please do something about the pain. This section will detail the medical approach to relieving this cruel form of pain. Its ramifications, of course, go far beyond the physical dimension, but I will say more about this later.

Unrelieved pain robs a person of quality time and may ultimately lead to despair and a sense of hopelessness. Family and friends are not spared, as they look on helplessly, wondering what can be done to relieve their relative/friend's suffering. Treatment of resistant pain is an urgent matter, not only because of the pain, but also to counteract the untold emotional harm that can result if the pain continues for any length of time.

In most cases, pain relief comes from using a larger dose of morphine. While this may be effective, it introduces a new set of problems, the main one being drowsiness. The choice is ultimately the patient's, and a trial of an increased dose is often the only way he/she can decide. The ultimate dose required to control the pain may be large, but a gradual increase rather than a sudden escalation allows adequate time for the doctor, patient and family to evaluate the benefits and side effects of treatment.

In some instances, side effects may be surprisingly minor, but for most people, drowsiness and confusion are the greatest concern. Drowsiness may be acceptable but confusion never is and a dose reduction may be required. If this compromises pain relief, the doctor will almost certainly change to a different analgesic.

You may hear or read reports that suggest large doses of an analgesic can hasten death by depressing respiration, thereby implying that this approach to pain relief is nothing short of euthanasia. These reports are misleading and alarmist and create unnecessary angst for all concerned. Analgesics used correctly do not hasten death. If you are worried about this, speak to the most senior doctor involved in your relative's/friend's care and discuss the matter fully.

When pain is severe, relief often comes at a cost. In the example that follows we see how communication, negotiation and careful planning can show the way.

Dawn had multiple myeloma, a malignancy that softens bones and increases the likelihood of fractures. She had several fractured ribs as a result of coughing. This caused considerable pain, particularly on movement. The only relief was from morphine but the dose required for relief resulted in drowsiness. Dawn chose to remain alert and only asked for extra morphine at night to help with sleep, or during the day when the pain was particularly severe.

She knew she was dying, but as there were several family rifts she chose to remain as alert as possible, hoping to heal these divisions. Despite the pain and discomfort she organised family meetings and presided over sessions that not only brought healing to the warring parties but also to herself. When this was completed she requested larger doses of morphine to ease the pain. The dose was increased until she was comfortable at rest, with only mild discomfort on turning and movement. She was drowsier than before, but was still able to maintain meaningful contact with her family until several days before her death.

Times like these can be particularly tough going. Accepting the death of someone you love is hard enough, but to witness suffering in the form of unrelieved pain, or to be asked to make compromises for the sake of pain relief, is challenging. If this is true for you, find someone you can talk to, someone who can hear your story without feeling they must solve the problem. If you have misgivings about the way your loved one's pain is being managed, ask for a meeting with the doctor(s) and nurses, let them know of your concerns and seek clarification about the treatment plan. This may not ease your immediate concern but advocating for your relative and taking positive steps to deal with uncertainty removes some of the helplessness and hopelessness that can otherwise overwhelm. It is the 'not knowing' that causes the most harm. The treatment of resistant pain may be problematic, but know there is always something that can be done.

Before outlining the options available (see below), I must stress that these alternatives are generally introduced after morphine and/or other analgesics have been given an adequate trial. The drugs mentioned are not used instead of morphine, but in combination with it. The response is variable and unpredictable and in most cases the search for the best treatment (or combination of treatments) is a matter of trial and error.

- Drugs other than conventional analgesics can sometimes help with resistant pain. These medications are grouped under the name 'co-analgesics' and in combination with conventional analgesics they may improve certain forms of pain, especially nerve pain. Co-analgesics include steroids (cortisone), ketamine (an anaesthetic agent) and drugs commonly used to treat conditions such as depression, epilepsy or heart troubles.
- A change in the type of analgesic may be recommended as each

works a little differently. So, if morphine has not been effective or is associated with intolerable side effects, another analgesic may give better results. Methadone is often recommended in this situation.

- A spinal infusion is occasionally recommended, but certain conditions need to be met before this can be considered. Morphine, in combination with other drugs, can be infused directly around the spinal cord where they act to relieve pain. Delivering medications directly to the point at which they act means the dose required for pain relief is much smaller than if they were given by mouth or injection. Consequently, side effects are less. Despite this theoretical advantage, a spinal infusion gives mixed results. It works well for some but not for others. Careful selection is the key to its success.
- In the very unusual situation where pain persists despite all measures, the option of sedation needs to be considered. Sedation does not eliminate pain but, as the person sleeps, they are less aware of it. This is a very complex situation and the use of sedation to ease pain has significant legal, moral and ethical implications. The decision is not taken lightly and is only implemented after full and open discussion. Family members often find the choice very hard to accept and derive little comfort from seeing their relative more asleep than awake, even though pain-free. We, in the medical profession, tread a fine line when we embark on this path, but we embark on it because, at this point, there are no alternatives. It is not, as some critics have suggested, a form of euthanasia. If done ethically and sensitively it is humane care of someone who would otherwise die in pain. The patients themselves say they fear dying in pain more than death itself.

The pain of dying

A chapter on pain would be incomplete without some mention of the anguish people feel when confronted with their imminent death. Even though I have worked in palliative care for twenty years, it is impossible for me to know what this might be like. Many of my dying patients say the experience is as indescribable as it is incomprehensible. Surreal is the word they most frequently come up with. If it is surreal for them, then it is impossible for us to know what they are feeling, for their pain is beyond our world and our understanding. As a North American Indian proverb says, 'In order to truly understand a man, one must walk a mile in his moccasins'.

Despite this, it is important to at least draw your attention to this very real source of suffering, which all dying people experience in their own unique way, and then to suggest ways you can be present for them.

Unlike physical pain, the pain of dying cannot be palliated by drugs. I would go so far as to say that drugs used to treat this form of pain ultimately do more harm than good, and that comforting measures are also counterproductive – the pain of dying is beyond the therapeutic reach of science and technology. Although it defies logic, the best thing you can the do is to allow your relative to talk about how they feel. Often it is hard for them to find the words, but sooner or later they will say something like, 'I didn't think it would be like this' or 'I don't want to die, but I can't live this way' or 'I don't want to leave you' or simply, 'I'm scared'. This is when you need to sit and listen. Silence, your presence and undivided attention is what they need at this time. The aim is not to try and make your loved one feel better, but to help them feel the pain that is deep inside. Once the confused and chaotic emotions that torment them are deeply felt (not necessarily understood) healing commences. Tears are always a good sign. Let me illustrate this with a true story.

> *Mavis had been admitted to the palliative care unit because of pain from advanced cancer. Her pain responded quickly to moderate doses of morphine, but depression, first noted on admission, became much worse. Counselling and anti-depressants made very little difference, and Mavis withdrew. She was unwilling (or unable) to talk to anyone. Reluctantly, she*

agreed to attend an art therapy class where the task that day was to draw an apple. Mavis quietly worked away in the corner of the room, and towards the end of the class she was seen to be crying. When the therapist went to check, he noted she had drawn an apple core rather than an apple. Later she revealed how the apple core image had allowed her to connect with her grief – grief about how the cancer was eating her away on the inside and destroying her life (the outside) at the same time.

Words are painfully inadequate when we attempt to describe the experience of dying. For this reason, metaphor or symbolism often becomes the only means by which a person can feel or express something that is otherwise ineffable. While they may struggle to tell you how they feel, a picture, a photo, a memory, a favourite tune or an image may, as was the case with Mavis, induce a wave of emotions that establishes a link between what they feel on the inside and what is happening to them on the outside. Once this connection is made, what was until then surreal becomes a little more real.

What then can you, as a carer, do if you see or feel your loved one's suffering? The answer may seem simple but is much harder to carry out than it sounds. When the moment arrives, allow them to experience their sorrow. Don't reassure, console, change the subject, get up to answer a phone or fabricate some reason to leave the room. Just be there for them. Asking questions is one sure way of getting them out of their heart and into their head, so don't feel as though you need to speak or make things better. Silence as always is golden.

Don't be deceived into thinking your role in all this is just one of a spectator. Your presence creates the space that allows all this to happen. It is as if you hold the light that allows your loved one to find their way. While your loved one will benefit from this intimate moment, you may need a friend or counsellor with whom you can debrief and let go of your own pain. As a carer, it is important that you also care for yourself

Chapter 4

Symptoms other than pain

Palliative care seeks to make
a person's body a comfortable
enough place to live in...

DR. RICHARD LAMERTON
Palliative Care Physician

Chapter 4

Symptoms other than pain

Time is precious for someone who is dying but it is the quality of that person's life that determines its value. The term 'quality of life' has become something of a cliché in palliative care, and while there is no strict definition, most would agree that bodily comfort is an essential ingredient. Those of you who have experienced severe pain and intractable vomiting or have gasped for air will appreciate how symptoms like these can undermine quality of life. Indeed it is not uncommon to hear a person burdened by one of these problems say, 'I wish I could die'. Of course we know this is not to be interpreted literally, but the comment says a lot for how physical discomfort impacts on life and living.

For most of us, symptoms that affect quality of life are usually transient. We are grateful when they subside and we go to great lengths to avoid a recurrence. Spare a thought then for those with a life-threatening illness whose symptoms are more distressing, and will persist unless adequately treated. A life of constant pain, nausea or breathlessness can drive the strongest person to despair.

It is for this reason palliative care places so much emphasis on the control and prevention of symptoms and the maintenance of the best possible quality of life. There is no hope of a cure for those referred to palliative care, but symptoms related to the underlying disease are generally amenable to treatment. No one should have to suffer unremitting physical distress and palliative care stakes its reputation on the ability to ease pain and many of the other symptoms that could otherwise make life intolerable. This chapter will look at the various ways palliative care can make the body of those with a life-threatening illness a comfortable enough place to live in.

While most of what follows is directed to carers, we must always remember that a patient is not a mere onlooker in the management of their illness or its symptoms. They need to be included, informed and empowered, for often the fear of the unknown and a sense of helplessness (lack of control) are ultimately more damaging to their psyche than any symptom is to their body. Control of the physical symptom is only part of what we, in palliative care, call holistic care.

Breathlessness

In the context of palliative care, breathlessness is most frequently seen in those with disease of the heart, lungs or kidneys, or with motor neuron disease, cancer of the lung or any other form of cancer that has spread to the lung. The resulting difficulty with breathing depends on the severity of the underlying disease and the presence or absence of other complicating factors such as anaemia, obesity, a chest infection, fluid around the lung (pleural effusion) or heart (pericardial effusion). Any one or a combination of these problems makes breathing harder, and it is this and the resulting shortage of oxygen that leads to the symptom of breathlessness.

The distress associated with breathlessness should never be underestimated. It can be very frightening, particularly during sudden or severe exacerbations, so much so the person may think they are about to die. Even though it is a highly visible symptom, the level of distress is often underestimated. So always rely on what your loved one says and if you are uncertain, ask your doctor or palliative care nurse to assess the situation.

The appropriateness and value of antibiotics in treating a chest infection will depend on circumstances other than the nature of the infection. As a general rule, the sicker the person and the closer they are to death, the less likely antibiotics will help. Having said this, the decision for or against antibiotics is never easy. I will say more about this in Chapter 9

If anaemia is present, the value of a blood transfusion has to be weighed up carefully. It occasionally helps, but in many cases the results are disappointing because there are other, more important, factors causing the breathlessness. Each case needs be considered on its merits, and the management of anaemia in the context of breathlessness should be discussed with your doctor. Much the same applies to the management of a pleural or pericardial effusion.

General measures to help breathlessness

- The most important thing you can do if your relative becomes breathless is stay with them. Breathlessness can be frightening, particularly if severe or if it is a relatively new feature of the illness. So avoid leaving them alone for any length of time. If you have to leave the room to ring for help or get medication, tell them, and return quickly. Your presence is reassuring and comforting, but you can also be of practical help by directing your relative to focus on their breathing. If it is possible, get them to take slower and deeper breaths.
- Those who are breathless generally prefer a well ventilated room. A stuffy, overheated room can make them feel worse even if it does not make breathing harder. A fan may also help.
- Oxygen is required in all but the mildest forms of breathlessness. The need for home oxygen should be discussed with the doctor

early in the course of the illness. If it is recommended, the doctor or community nurse will make the necessary arrangements for its delivery and they or the supplier will show you how to use the equipment. I will say more about oxygen shortly but, on a practical note, oxygen concentrators (not cylinders) are available free of charge to those who are linked to a palliative care program.

- Plan ahead so that activities that induce breathlessness, such as showering and toileting, are well spaced.
- For those who use oxygen intermittently, ten minutes of oxygen before exertion can be helpful. If oxygen is used continuously, increasing the flow rate may be of some benefit. Plan any activities mindfully and proceed in an unhurried way.
- Take whatever measures are necessary to prevent constipation as this sets up a vicious cycle where constipation aggravates breathlessness and vice versa.

Oxygen

Oxygen is a virtual lifeline for those who are breathless, and when required is administered via nasal prongs or face mask. The nasal route is usually the better and preferred option. It interferes less with eating, is not as claustrophobic as a mask and poses less of a barrier to communication. Oxygen is run at 2–3 litres/minute when given via prongs and 4–5 litres/minute by mask.

The commonest source of home oxygen is an oxygen concentrator. This is a mains operated machine that plugs into your normal three-point plug. When switched on it extracts oxygen from the atmosphere and concentrates the gas in a reservoir. The concentrator makes a constant droning noise, which some people find irritating. This is easily overcome by placing the concentrator in another room and running a long connection (supplied at the time of delivery) to the prongs or mask. Unlike oxygen via a cylinder, concentrators provide an endless supply of oxygen – most deliver a maximum of 5 litres/minute, but some of the newer models manage 8 litres/minute. Running at the maximum rate for prolonged periods can overwork the machine and result in mechanical problems. Oxygen via nasal prongs can cause the lining of the nose to become very dry, resulting in nose bleeds. This can be addressed by keeping the flow rate at 2 litres/minute or by applying Vaseline to the nostrils. If these measures fail, a humidifier, available from the oxygen supplier, will moisten the inspired oxygen and lessen the problem.

Oxygen can be given at much higher rates (up to 10–12 litres/minute) via a cylinder, but the hiring and replacement costs of cylinders and the associated logistics make this a less attractive alternative. The concentrator is usually the preferred option. It is easy to use, very effective and the 'quality' of the oxygen it delivers is as good as that from a cylinder. Although concentrators are very reliable, blackouts still occur, and for this reason a backup supply of oxygen is recommended in many cases not only to deal with power failure, but also to facilitate short outings from home.

Oxygen is highly inflammable and should not be used near an open flame or where sparks could occur. Smoking should, of course, be prohibited within the home.

Morphine

Morphine is also used to treat breathlessness. This may come as a surprise but morphine and oxygen are two of the most effective agents for the treatment of this distressing symptom. Morphine is generally given by mouth and experience suggests the liquid (quick-acting form) is more effective than the slow-release tablet or capsule. If breathlessness is intermittent or mild, the medication may be used only as required. In other cases it is usual for the morphine to be given regularly (as it is for pain) with extra or breakthrough doses for exacerbations (see Chapter 3 for further details on breakthrough morphine). If required, the dose of morphine can be increased, just as it is for pain.

Occasionally, morphine is administered via a nebuliser even though evidence suggests it is no better than morphine by mouth. If the nebulised route is recommended, be aware it is injectable morphine that is used; the liquid or oral form cannot be used in a nebuliser.

Some doctors are a little hesitant about using morphine to treat breathlessness, particularly in the face of emphysema. Their concern arises from teaching that once said morphine could aggravate rather than improve breathlessness resulting from chronic lung conditions. Subsequent research has shown this to be incorrect and has irrefutably confirmed that morphine, if used correctly, is safe and one of the best treatments for breathlessness, irrespective of the cause.

Benzodiazepines

This class of drugs, of which Valium® (diazepam) is the best known example, may be helpful in situations where breathlessness continues to be troublesome despite the optimum use of morphine and oxygen. Small doses of a benzodiazepine called lorazepam (Ativan®) may be given once or twice daily in the hope of improving sleep as well as relieving breathlessness.

Steroids

'Steroid' is a generic name for a group of drugs that have an anti-inflammatory effect. You may be more familiar with the term cortisone – for the sake of this discussion cortisone and steroids are considered one and the same thing. Steroids are often useful for inflammatory conditions, particularly if there is associated swelling. We all know how useful they can be for asthma, but they can also help those whose breathlessness results from cancer compressing one of the bronchi (breathing tubes) or if the cancer has invaded the lymphatic tissue in the substance and surface of the lung (lymphangitis). The steroids most commonly prescribed for these conditions are dexamethasone, prednisone and prednisolone. If steroids do help, the benefit usually follows within days and may last for weeks or months. Steroids occasionally benefit those with emphysema, and a trial of treatment is often recommended by doctors.

Steroids have well known side-effects that tend to appear after a period of use exceeding 2 to 4 weeks. These include a fungal infection of the mouth and throat (thrush), difficulty with sleeping, particularly if the steroid is taken late in the day, facial swelling, increased facial hair in women, a tendency to bruise easily, ankle swelling and weakness of the muscles around the hips and shoulders. Steroids can also exacerbate pre-existing nervous conditions and elevate the blood pressure and blood sugar levels. Care should therefore be exercised if they are prescribed to those with a psychiatric history, hypertension and diabetes mellitus.

Radiotherapy

Radiotherapy has a very limited role in the treatment of breathlessness resulting from cancer. It is generally reserved for those whose cancer is compressing one of the larger airways. The effect of radiotherapy is to shrink the cancer, permitting air to move more freely through the airway. Radiotherapy can also be used to treat cancer within the substance of the lung. This is never a straightforward matter, so the final decision generally rests with the radiotherapist.

Surgical procedures

There are now some surgical procedures and interventions that have been tried and found to benefit a small group of people with breathlessness. They are not commonly performed, but this could change as technology improves and the procedures are simplified. I will mention just two:

stenting for lung cancer and lung reduction surgery for emphysema. For more information you should speak to your doctor.

What can you do for a severe episode of breathlessness?

- If oxygen is in the home but not in use, connect it up immediately and run it at maximum capacity (5 litres/minute for a concentrator; 8–10 litres/minute for a cylinder).
- If the oxygen is already in use, check that it is turned up to the maximum flow rate and that there are no blockages in the system – usually there is a whistling noise if the tubing is blocked. Make sure all the connections are firm. If you have a cylinder, ensure it is not empty.
- Sit the person upright and open nearby windows.
- If your relative/friend has morphine as part of their regular medication, give a breakthrough dose.
- Ring the doctor and/or nurse.
- Sit with the person until help arrives.
- Do not leave your relative/friend for extended periods of time.
- With the help of your doctor or nurse, develop a plan to cope with possible future attacks.

Stridor

Stridor is the name given to croup-like breathing that occasionally accompanies some neck and lung cancers. This whistling or high-pitched noise occurs when cancer presses on and narrows one of the larger airways. The sound is heard during inspiration and expiration, and is usually present throughout the day and night. It may be accompanied by a feeling of breathlessness and a dry cough. The combination of stridor and breathlessness can be distressing for the patient and the carer, and not uncommonly exacerbates or induces a fear of suffocating. With good palliative care this should never occur. If you have cause for concern, speak to your doctor or nurse.

Cough

In the palliative care situation a cough is commonly associated with cancer of the lung, emphysema and severe heart failure. With cancer, the cough is often persistent with little or no associated sputum. Occasionally, streaks of bright red blood will be present in the sputum and sometimes the amount can be surprisingly large. If there is a lot of blood, notify the doctor or nurse immediately. Rarely will anything need to be done, but if bleeding occurs frequently or if the volume of blood increases, a change in medication or radiotherapy may be recommended.

Coughing of blood also occurs with heart failure, blood clots and some chest infections. Reporting it to the doctor allows him/her to consider all the possibilities and the best treatment.

In the absence of blood, simple measures such as a cough mixture may be all that is required. If this fails and the cough is distressing, morphine in small doses is very effective. Morphine is generally given by mouth but this is one of the few occasions when it may be as effective via a nebuliser, with or without Ventolin®.

A cough with small or copious amounts of sputum is the norm with emphysema. Cough suppressants are best avoided as they increase the risk of sputum retention and a chest infection, both of which could have serious consequences. The sputum, in this case, is better out than in.

Nausea and vomiting

These two symptoms are particularly prominent in people with kidney failure, cancer of the stomach, colon and pancreas, as well as cancer that has spread to the liver. Both symptoms are distressing, even when they occur in an otherwise healthy individual, and this distress is proportionally greater in those who are already weakened from the effects of serious illness. Apart from the underlying illness there are other factors that may cause or aggravate nausea and vomiting. These need to be considered and excluded, particularly if the symptoms do not respond to standard treatment. These factors include:

- constipation. This is one of the commonest and most overlooked causes of nausea and vomiting and must be excluded in all cases
- blockage in the bowel. In this case the symptoms are due to a mechanical obstruction, usually from cancer (see below)
- mouth infections, including thrush
- poor kidney function
- excess calcium in the blood. This is confirmed by a blood test, and if elevated, specific treatment is available to lower the calcium, which in turn improves the symptoms
- medications including morphine, antibiotics, anti-inflammatory drugs, diuretics (fluid tablets) and some laxatives. When medication is thought to be the cause, your doctor will probably withdraw the offending drug(s) and substitute it with an acceptable alternative. If the drug is essential, it will be continued and an anti-emetic introduced
- overfeeding. This is an uncommon cause but should be considered when all of the above have been excluded. It often results from an overly concerned relative encouraging their loved one to eat more than they really want (see section on weight loss in Chapter 5)
- a combination of any of the above.

Nausea and vomiting secondary to a bowel blockage from cancer present a challenging problem. No amount of anti-vomiting medication is likely to eliminate the symptoms entirely, and surgery is often not possible, especially if the person is too weak and unwell or if the cancer is advanced. While medication may not stop the vomiting, it reduces the frequency. Despite the blockage, a small amount of fluids can still be taken by mouth to ease thirst. This is unlikely to aggravate the vomiting providing due care is taken with the type of fluid and the volume. Water and other clear fluids (lemonade) are tolerated best. Fluid replacement via a 'drip' may or may not have a place.

Food intake is virtually a non-issue. Those with a bowel blockage have little or no desire to eat and can barely tolerate the sight or smell of food. It is not uncommon in this situation for families to worry that not eating or drinking will result in death from starvation or dehydration. Death in this setting is inevitable and does not result from lack of food or fluid, but from the widespread effects of cancer (see Chapter 5 for further information). Attempts at feeding in this situation are almost always counterproductive and further impair the quality of life.

Finally, some mention should be made of cancer in the liver. There is a widely held belief that death follows quickly once cancer has spread to the liver. This is not altogether true, as the outcome depends more on the type of cancer and how fast it is growing than on the liver involvement itself. The liver is a remarkable organ and can continue to function for quite a long time even when much of it has been replaced by cancer. Some people can live for many months or longer despite liver involvement by cancer.

Medications used to improve nausea and vomiting

Numerous medications can be used to prevent or treat nausea and vomiting. These are called anti-emetics. The most popular and commonly used anti-emetics are as follows (generic name followed by brand name):

- haloperidol (Serenace®)
- metoclopramide (Maxolon®)
- domperidone (Motilium®)
- prochlorperazine (Stemetil®)
- promethazine (Phenergan®)
- corticosteroids (Dexamethasone®)
- ondansetron (Zofran®).

Anti-emetics are generally given by mouth unless vomiting is intractable, when they are given by injection under the skin to ensure adequate absorption. Depending on the cause, the doctor will initiate treatment with one of the anti-emetics listed above. This is successful in the majority of instances. If not, the doctor has several options:

- increase the dose
- use a different anti-emetic
- use a combination of anti-emetics
- give the anti-emetic by injection.

Anti-emetics are prescribed to control and prevent vomiting, so they are given regularly and continued even when the vomiting has settled. To withdraw treatment at that point may lead to a return of symptoms. As is the case with most drugs, anti-emetics are not free of side effects. They may cause drowsiness or result in a measure of restlessness. In either case the medication will be changed or the dose reduced. Most of these medications can also aggravate Parkinson's disease and due caution is exercised when choosing an anti-emetic in this situation.

Difficulty with swallowing (dysphagia)

Dysphagia literally means pain with swallowing. If pain is the major problem, particularly if it is localised to the throat, thrush is a very likely cause. For further information, see 'Mouth care' in Chapter 5. In the absence of thrush, difficulty with swallowing may be due to a blockage in the oesophagus, often but not always from cancer. In this case, dysphagia is worse with solids and the person will say food gets stuck, and will indicate the spot by pointing to the lower neck or to the front of the chest.

If dysphagia is due to cancer, the patient and family face the difficult decision of pursuing invasive, but potentially life-prolonging treatment or opting for no treatment other than supportive/palliative care. It is a veritable cross road in the life of the patient. The implications for life and death are clear. The palliative approach is more likely when the person is clearly dying, but life-prolonging treatment is more appropriate for someone who still has a good quality of life. The story, however, is different when there is uncertainty about prognosis. In all cases the final choice will ultimately rest with the patient, but an informed decision is only possible when all possible options have been fully discussed.

In such a highly charged situation, disagreement is not uncommon – some family members will want active treatment while others will feel the time has come for comfort measures only. Consensus may or may not be achieved but it is important that everyone has the opportunity to express an opinion. A meeting with the doctor, the patient and significant family can sometimes resolve any impasse and prevent long-term family rifts.

A full discussion of treatment options is beyond the scope of this book but possible interventions for dysphagia due to cancer of the oesophagus include:

- radiotherapy (with or without chemotherapy) to shrink the cancer. The course of radiotherapy is often prolonged and the dysphagia usually gets worse before it gets better. For this reason a PEG (percutaneous endoscopic gastrostomy) tube (see below) may be inserted beforehand
- placement of a stent inside the oesophagus to widen the lumen and improve swallowing
- insertion of a feeding or PEG tube to provide an alternative route (other than by mouth) for nutritional fluids to be administered. The tube opens into the stomach and the other end exits via the abdominal wall, thus bypassing the blockage. A PEG tube may be used in conjunction with radiotherapy or alone when it represents a palliative approach to care
- subcutaneous fluids as a temporary palliative option.

For further information on any of these, speak to your doctor or community nurse. If a decision is made not to intervene, treatment follows the course outlined under 'Fluids' in Chapter 5.

Loss of appetite

See Chapter 5, 'Day-to-day care'.

Constipation

See Chapter 5, 'Day-to-day care'.

Fatigue and weakness

Loss of appetite, loss of weight and loss of energy are frequent accompaniments of any life-threatening illness and ultimately render people so weak they eventually require assistance with most activities of daily living. The degree of weakness often (but not always) parallels the rate and degree of weight loss. If this is the case, you would imagine good meals and/or protein supplements would reverse the weakness or stop it from getting worse. Sadly, it doesn't. Even if a person's intake is adequate, they are unable to process food in the usual way and much of the food's nutritional value is lost. This all results from the underlying disease and is a well recognised complication of cancer. Many other factors such as inactivity, medication, depression, anaemia and pre-existing health problems also contribute to the weakness and fatigue, but their role is relatively small in comparison to that of the underlying disease.

According to many surveys, weakness and fatigue are two of the most distressing and disabling symptoms found in those who are dying. Unlike other symptoms such as pain, breathlessness, nausea and vomiting, there is little useful treatment. Not only do they result in loss of independence, they also increase the risk of complications such as falls and pressure areas. The overall effect on the person's quality of life is quite marked. Although there is no specific treatment, I will offer a few suggestions:

- Allow the person to do as little or as much as they want. Encouraging unrealistic activity in someone who is weak is not physically or psychologically helpful and may compromise safety.

- Loss of independence is a major consequence of weakness. It can have profound physical and psychological repercussions. Equipment and home aids may facilitate independence, improve dignity, self worth and safety. An occupational therapist can advise you about home aids and the best and safest way to care for your loved one at home.
- If you suspect depression is contributing to the inactivity, ask the doctor to assess the situation and advise on the relative merits of anti-depressant medication and general supportive measures.
- If the person is anaemic, blood transfusion rarely makes a difference and is inappropriate if death is near. If the person is not so ill, treatment of anaemia may be helpful if the physical deterioration corresponds with the onset of anaemia. In most cases, however, the overall benefits of transfusion in those with advanced disease is somewhat disappointing. Consider the matter carefully and discuss management with the doctor if anaemia is found to be present.

Before leaving this subject, I must mention one uncommon but potentially treatable cause of weakness, namely spinal cord compression. This happens when cancer in or around the spine presses on the spinal cord, leading to the relatively rapid onset of weakness in both legs. This may or may not be accompanied by back pain, numbness in the legs and difficulty with passing urine. If any of these symptoms occur, the doctor or nurse should be notified immediately as treatment with steroids, radiotherapy and, in some instances, surgery, can prevent progression and may even lead to partial or full recovery.

Hiccups

Although they are an infrequent complication of illness, hiccups are distressing, particularly if they are persistent. They occur in renal failure, with irritation to the diaphragm from cancer or because of a full stomach secondary to a bowel obstruction. Careful attention to the quantity and frequency of fluid intake may improve the situation if a bowel obstruction is present. Otherwise, the usual tricks, such as swallowing granulated sugar or holding one's breath can be tried, but rarely work in the context of advanced illness. If the problem is ongoing, medication is often required. Again, there is no guarantee of success. Your doctor will advise on the relative merits of possible treatments, which include metoclopramide (Maxolon®) or baclofen (Lioresal®). The latter is often successful if all others have failed, but it can aggravate tiredness.

Ascites

Ascites is a swelling of the abdomen that occurs when fluid accumulates inside the abdominal cavity. It occurs with certain cancers, cirrhosis of the liver and occasionally with heart failure. The swelling may be minor or so marked it resembles a 'full term pregnancy'. Not only is the abdomen visibly distended, it is also distinctly uncomfortable, resulting in fullness, bloating, reflux, breathlessness and moderate to severe pain. Often there is associated swelling of the ankles and lower legs.

The presence of fluid can be confirmed by examination, but an ultrasound is sometimes required. If drainage is recommended, this is usually done in hospital, a palliative care ward or occasionally in the person's home. Drainage is a simple, painless and relatively safe procedure. A cannula (very similar to the one used for a drip) is inserted through the anaesthetised skin of the abdomen. This is advanced until fluid begins to drain. A tube is attached to the cannula and the ascitic fluid runs into a drainage bag. The volume that drains may be as small as 1 litre or as much as 10 litres. The duration of the procedure varies, but rarely extends beyond a few hours. The person may sit in a chair or remain in bed while the ascites is draining.

Ascites is drained only if the associated symptoms warrant, and relief is then immediate. The fluid is rich in protein and the major drawback to the procedure is the loss of this valuable source of nutrition. For this reason, the procedure is only performed if symptoms warrant and not merely because fluid is noted. The relief is unfortunately temporary as the ascites invariably re-accumulates, often requiring a repeat drainage within weeks or months. Drainage may aggravate pre-existing fatigue and weakness but this improves spontaneously over the following days and is helped by encouraging the person to drink. Reducing the fluid intake does not prevent or reduce the rate at which the ascites re-accumulates and will only make weakness and a dry mouth worse. Fluid tablets may be of some use in managing the ascites if it is due to liver or heart disease, but rarely helps when cancer is the cause.

Confusion

Confusion or, to be more exact, delirium can occur in those who are nearing the end of life. Confusion manifests in numerous ways but most frequently as disturbed thinking, disorientation, seemingly unconnected thoughts and agitation. Inappropriate behaviour is also common and may be one of the earliest signs. This includes such things as looking at a book upside down, pouring tea into the milk jug, aimless wandering and urinary incontinence. The earliest signs can be so subtle as to be missed and, not uncommonly, appear after sunset – darkness is known to exacerbate confusion.

The confused person often has some insight into their problem and may have periods of lucidity when they feel embarrassed about what they have done or the inconvenience they have caused. Your gentle messages of love and under-standing will go a long way towards comforting and reassuring them as well as settling the delirium, albeit temporarily.

While delirium may be an inevitable accompaniment of illness and dying, the reason for its appearance is complex and often related to a combination of factors. In the context of cancer, however, two questions invariably arise: Is the delirium due to morphine? Has the cancer spread to the brain?

Is the delirium due to morphine?

Morphine (or any other opioids for that matter) may cause or contribute to delirium and the likelihood increases as the dose is escalated. So delirium secondary to analgesics should be considered when a large dose is currently in use or when the onset of delirium is closely related to the commencement of the opioid or to an increase in its dose. As delirium caused by opioids is almost always dose-related, an appropriate dose reduction often improves the situation without compromising pain relief. Reductions are made slowly and incrementally as a rapid reduction could result in an exacerbation of pain. Rather than reduce the dose, your doctor may change to another opioid, for delirium is often drug specific – meaning it may occur with one opioid and not another.

I would not like to leave you with the idea that morphine (or other opioids) is the commonest cause of delirium in palliative care patients. It may be the first cause the doctor thinks of, but only because it is the easiest to treat. Other causes of delirium or factors that contribute to its onset include infection, other drugs, vitamin deficiency, frequent changes in the sensory environment (over stimulation), under stimulation, lack of quality sleep, unremitting pain, alterations in the blood chemistry, and low blood sugar levels (in diabetics).

Many of these causes of delirium can be treated, but the decision to do so depends as much on the proximity to death as it does on the level of confusion. Comfort measures are more appropriate when death is near, but for those with a reasonable prognosis, investigation, reversal of complicating factors and appropriate treatment is warranted.

Has the cancer spread to the brain?

Contrary to popular belief, a 'brain' tumour is a relatively uncommon cause of delirium, irrespective of whether it has arisen in or spread to the brain. Brain tumours can cause delirium but it is not an automatic association.

In other words, if a person with a brain tumour becomes confused, other causes need to be considered before the confusion is attributed to the tumour. How actively this line of investigation is pursued (if at all) will depend on the overall state of the person concerned more than the degree of confusion. If the person is unwell and close to death, investigation is unlikely to alter the outcome and efforts aimed at maintaining comfort and dignity will ultimately be more beneficial. The situation is different with those who are less sick, as Isabel's case illustrates.

> *Isabel was in her early sixties and had a very rapidly growing cancer that had spread to her bones. She was depressed and had quite a lot of pain that ultimately improved with morphine. Over four to eight weeks her husband had noticed minor but uncharacteristic changes in her behaviour and thinking. He was prompted to report these only after Isabel attempted to get out of a moving car. Examination and tests revealed no obvious cause for the delirium and the situation did not improve after the morphine dose was reduced. A brain scan did not show a definite tumour although there were some changes that suggested the cancer had spread to the linings of the brain.*
>
> *Isabel was admitted to the local hospice with a view to investigating and treating the delirium. As is customary, all medication that seemed unnecessary was ceased at the time of admission. Within days there was a small but significant improvement in Isabel's mental state, and after one week she was virtually back to normal. A review of her previous medication led us to conclude the delirium was due to an anti-depressant drug that had been commenced just before the delirium was noted. The diagnosis was confirmed after a search of the medical literature showed that this drug did indeed cause delirium, albeit rarely.*

Palliative care patients are more susceptible to the side effects of most medications. So if delirium should occur, ask the doctor to review the treatment and, where possible, to reduce the dose of those medications that must be continued and stop those no longer necessary.

What can you do to improve delirium?

- If the person is confused about time and place, orientate them as often as is necessary by telling them where they are and what is happening. A friend of mine died recently. Prior to her death she was confused, and this was clearly as distressing to her as it was to those who knew her. I got into the habit of orientating her whenever I visited. I introduced myself, told her the time of day and the day of the week. I took nothing for granted. I explained what I was about to do (e.g. feed her), identified any noise that took her attention (e.g. washing machine, outside traffic) and told her who else was in the house. This not only helped to orientate her, but also had a marked effect in reducing her restlessness.
- Keep familiar photos and favourite objects nearby and play music they know and like.
- Keep the environment as constant as possible. Sensory overload with lots of different visitors or frequent changes of scenery can add to the confusion.
- Be aware of safety issues – for example, do not leave dangerous items nearby, supervise the drinking of hot fluids, take care with heaters.
- Delirium is often worse at night – familiar background music and a soft night-light may help.
- If the delirium is marked, a roster may need to be drawn up to ensure a familiar face is always present.
- If all these measures have been tried and the delirium is persistent,

distressing, undignified or potentially dangerous, medication may be required. There are several treatment options and your doctor will speak to you about them.

Fitting

Fitting occurs a little more frequently in the palliative care population. Fitting is distressing for all concerned and often provokes anxiety in the carer who, faced with a potential crisis, may be frightened and uncertain of how best to respond.

Most people are familiar with or would recognise the most common fit, the so called 'grand mal'. With this, the person's body stiffens and this is followed by jerking or shaking movements that involve the whole body, but are most obvious in the arms and legs. The fit may be as short as a few seconds or as long as several minutes. During this time, breathing is noisy, skin colour changes from pink to a bluish hue and there may be incontinence of urine and faeces. The person is unconscious throughout the episode and for some time after, and will therefore have no recollection of the event. When the shaking stops, as it invariably does, the person may sleep for a short time and breathing and colour gradually return to normal. When the person 'awakes' he/she may be confused for a brief period so it is important to reassure them, as they are often aware that something has happened.

In the event of a grand mal fit, the following measures are recommended:

- Do not attempt to restrain the person while they are shaking as this can result in damage to their muscles and ligaments.
- Do not attempt to put a peg or any other object between the teeth. This is impossible and unnecessary, and any attempt may break teeth or dislodge dentures.
- If they are in bed ensure, as best you can, they do not fall to the floor, otherwise leave them as you find them and use pillows or

blankets to prevent their head, arms or legs hitting against hard objects.

- If the person does not regain consciousness immediately after the fit has ceased, lay them on their side and remove any dentures. This will ensure they maintain a good airway and do not 'swallow their tongue'.
- Commence oxygen after the fit has stopped or earlier if the fit is prolonged. (This is not essential so do not be concerned if you do not have oxygen in the home.)
- Notify a doctor or nurse and then sit by the person until help arrives.
- It is not essential to ring an ambulance. However, this may be necessary if a second fit follows or if a doctor is unable to attend.
- When the person wakes, explain what has happened and reassure them that everything is now under control. This is particularly important if the person is confused.

Sometimes the fit may be partial with the shaking confined to one side of the body or parts thereof. There is no loss of consciousness with this type of fit, and colour and breathing remain unchanged. Reassurance is particularly important in this instance, as the person is fully aware of what is happening, is likely to be frightened and may even wonder if they are about to die. Again, the doctor or palliative care nurse should be notified.

Whether it is a full blown or partial fit, medication to prevent further fits is necessary. This is usually in tablet or capsule form but an injection may be given in the first instance. Depending on the state of health of the person and their anticipated life expectancy, investigations may or may not be required to determine the cause of the fitting.

Fits are not an invariable consequence of brain tumours. For this reason treatment to prevent them is rarely given when a brain tumour is diagnosed unless, of course, there has been a previous history of fitting. There are a few exceptions to this rule. Some 'brain' tumours are more prone to cause fits and it is not unusual for anti-convulsant medication to be given prophylactically in these situations. If your relative/friend has a tumour within the brain, ask the doctor about the need for medication to prevent fits or to have in the house in case of an emergency.

Ankle swelling

Oedema, or swelling of the ankles and legs, occurs in those with heart, liver or kidney failure and will appear at some stage in the course of cancer. In the later stages of cancer the swelling is often secondary to weight loss or other nutritional changes that occur around this time. Blood clots (deep vein thrombosis) are relatively common in those who are sick, particularly if they are confined to bed or a chair, and may at times be responsible for swelling.

Whatever the cause, protein-rich fluid accumulates under the skin and causes the swelling. It is first seen in the feet and around the ankles, gradually extending upwards and, in the severest form, may involve legs and the lower trunk. Pain does not normally accompany the swelling but the legs may be tender to touch. When pain is present, a blood clot is possible and may require specific treatment. If the swelling is marked, heaviness of the legs can be a problem. The added weight makes it harder for the person to lift their legs, get out of a chair or walk. It not only limits activity, it also compromises independence and introduces safety issues.

The skin over the swollen areas is often tissue paper thin and can tear with the slightest trauma. These tears may be microscopic or large and allow the oedema to seep out, resulting in dampness of clothing and bed linen. If this occurs, the area should be bandaged to contain the seepage and also to protect against further skin damage. The protein-rich fluid is a favourite culture medium for many bugs and due care must be taken to prevent infection, especially if a tear is present.

Elevating the legs helps to redistribute the fluid to other parts of the body and explains why ankle swelling improves after a night in bed and is worse after prolonged sitting or standing. For this reason it is helpful to keep the legs elevated when the person is sitting, but don't insist if this is too uncomfortable. Massage can also redistribute the fluid. This must be done carefully, bearing in mind the delicate state of the skin. Creams or oils that maintain skin integrity are also beneficial.

Elastic stockings may help to reduce swelling in those who are up and about. Stockings may be hot in summer and uncomfortable, so the potential benefits need to be weighed against these disadvantages. Fluid tablets are occasionally prescribed to reduce swelling, but their success rate is low and the incidence of side effects high. For this reason they are reserved for the 'relatively well' and even in that group great care must to be taken in the choice and dose of medication.

Sweating

Sweating can be a troublesome symptom in anyone who is unwell. It may be due to infection, a side effect of medication (morphine and paracetamol are the main offenders) or the illness itself (particularly lymphoma, leukaemia and widespread cancer). The sweats are more likely to occur at night, are frequently drenching and often require a change of pyjamas and bed linen. Treatment involves looking for and treating any cause (if appropriate) as well as the following comfort measures:

- Ensure the room is not too hot.
- Open windows or use a fan to circulate the air.
- Avoid warm clothing and too many blankets.
- Encourage the use of cotton pyjamas and bed linen, as cotton is less likely to induce sweating.
- Encourage the person to drink ample fluids.

In cases where the sweating is profuse and the above measures fail to offer relief, several medications have been trialled with varying degrees of success. Your doctor can tell you more about the relative merits of such treatment.

Infections

Patients with cancer of the lung, a history of chest troubles such as emphysema and those confined to bed are prone to chest infections. The infection manifests in the usual way with a fever, moist cough and coloured sputum, but occasionally these features are absent and the only tell-tale sign may be a sudden deterioration in the person's health.

Other sites of infection include the skin, bladder, kidney and blood. Skin infections or abscesses may occur around pressure areas or at the site of a previous injection or 'butterfly' needle. Bladder and kidney infections are more common in those with urinary catheters or with a previous history of similar infections. Cancer in the pelvic region, for example prostate cancer in men and cervical, uterine or ovarian cancer in women, may also predispose to kidney or bladder infections.

Blood infection (septicaemia) is generally seen in the very sick, those with leukaemia or lymphoma and those who are jaundiced. As with pneumonia, septicaemia can lead to a sudden and dramatic deterioration.

Most infections are treated with an appropriate antibiotic. Depending on the site of the infection, other measures may be necessary. For example, a skin abscess may need to be drained, a butterfly needle changed if the surrounding skin is swollen, and a urinary catheter removed or replaced if it is thought to be the cause of a kidney or bladder infection.

The use of antibiotics in someone close to death is another matter. Treatment at this time may be futile and inappropriate. I do not wish to imply that antibiotic treatment should never be given to someone who is dying, but only that the decision should be weighed carefully and guided by the known or expressed wish of that person as well as their state of health.

Itch (pruritis)

Itch is often present in those who are jaundiced, especially if the jaundice is due to a blockage to the flow of bile. This commonly occurs with cancer of the pancreas or cancer of the bile duct and in these cases, the deeper the jaundice the worse the itch. At its worst, the itch may cause marked restlessness and insomnia. The best treatment, if the person is well enough, is to relieve the jaundice and, depending on circumstances, this may involve surgery or inserting a stent in the bile duct.

A stent is a semi-rigid tube that is inserted through and beyond the obstruction, permitting the normal flow of bile to resume, thereby relieving the jaundice. The procedure does not require an operation. It is done endoscopically (by way of an endoscope – the same instrument used to inspect the inside of the stomach) and under light sedation. This is much simpler and less risky than surgery, but the benefits are temporary for stents are prone to blockage and infection. In these instances the old stent is removed and a new one reinserted, but each successive procedure becomes harder and ultimately impossible. Surgery gives a longer lasting result but is often too dangerous a proposition for those with advanced cancer.

If the person is too sick for either of these procedures or if the itch is due to another cause, such as lymphoma, soothing lotions and anti-histamines are the best options. Night sedation may overcome the associated sleep disturbance, but it is not uncommon to see people scratching even during sleep. Heat makes the itch worse, so any reasonable measures to address this may help.

Itch may also result from the use of morphine and may appear as part of an allergic reaction to certain drugs, particularly antibiotics. An alternative pain reliever to morphine or a change of antibiotics resolves these problems promptly.

A drug called cholestyramine (Questran®) is sometimes used when itch from jaundice cannot be palliated by other medications, surgery or stenting. It comes as powder and needs to be taken three or four times a day. It has an unpleasant taste, is constipating, and from my experience rarely gives worthwhile results

Bleeding

Bleeding from the bowel, bladder, lungs or other sites can be a source of concern, particularly if it occurs for the first time or if the blood loss is heavy. Bleeding is rarely accompanied by other symptoms, but fatigue, pallor and sweating may be present. Blood loss should always be reported to your doctor or nurse and the degree of urgency will depend on the volume lost and the physical and emotional state of your loved one. The presence of small amounts (streaks or spots) is much less significant, but it too should be reported as a matter of routine, though not urgently. If bleeding occurs, it is recommended that you discuss the possibility of further episodes with the doctor and develop a plan of action. See the end of this chapter for more information.

Insomnia

Difficulty with sleeping is not unique to those who are ill. Evidence suggests, however, that the quality of their sleep, irrespective of the amount, is often poor in this group of people. Pain, bodily discomfort, breathlessness and other symptoms contribute to this problem. Noise, a different bed and an unfamiliar environment are major factors for those in hospital or a palliative care unit. Fear of dying in one's sleep, fear of the future and existential crises may contribute and are often overlooked.

Physical and emotional problems always seem worse when we are alone, and a night without sleep is no exception. For those who are dying, a sleepless night may open Pandora's Box – thoughts and emotions go round and round, adding to the person's distress and making sleep even less likely. The loneliness of dying, the sadness of leaving those they love, uncertainty about the future, the fear of suffering, the thought of dying that night – all loom large and become more sinister in the long dark hours. It is no wonder those who are ill dread the night and a lack of sleep.

While all this may sound bad, it can also be seen as an opportunity for healing. This may seem unlikely, but the following example could help to illustrate my point.

> *Barbara had been admitted to the hospice because of pain from widespread cancer. She was in her early forties and happily married with one teenage daughter. According to her family, she had until then managed reasonably well at home, showing few signs of emotional distress. She had the occasional episode of panic, often while in the bathroom, but only when the door was shut. She had overcome this quite simply by leaving the bathroom door ajar.*
>
> *Pain medication was adjusted and after several days Barbara had little if any daytime pain and was seen to be fairly active around the ward. The nights were a different story. She was unable to sleep 'because of pain' and requested regular breakthrough doses of morphine. According to the night staff, this resulted in short periods of sleep but pain was always present when she woke 1 to 2 hours later.*
>
> *The night staff felt there was more behind the wakefulness than pain, and spent more time with her when she woke at night. As they talked, Barbara slowly opened up and spoke of her anxiety, her fear of dying, her concern for her family and how she was unlikely to complete many of the things she had planned for her future. During these outpourings Barbara did not complain of pain, and more often than not would go to sleep without the need for pain medication or sedation. After several nights Barbara's insomnia had all but resolved. She required no extra pain medication and slept for long periods throughout the night.*

While the night may bring darkness it, paradoxically, puts the spotlight on all the fears and concerns that have been neatly tucked away. Daytime activities are very effective in keeping emotions at bay, but these emotions often well up at night and catch us by surprise. In Barbara's case the worsening pain carried a strong message that the cancer was getting worse. This raised many fears and concerns which she managed to suppress while at home, even though the episodes of panic suggested they were very close to the surface.

In the unfamiliar hospice situation, with no husband to comfort her at night, Barbara was helpless to fend off the emotions that welled up during those long dark hours. What she called 'pain' was not physical pain but suffering and, not surprisingly, morphine did little to help. The brief periods of sleep simply put everything on hold until she woke, and when she did the 'demons' were still there. Desmond Tutu, in his book *No Future Without Forgiveness*, says, 'unless you look the beast in the eye you will find that it returns to hold you hostage'.

Talking about fears and concerns is one way of confronting the beasts and, in the case of insomnia, is often a more fruitful way of dealing with the problem than resorting to sedation or 'pain' relief. At times, sedation may be useful and necessary, but care must be taken to ensure the cause of the insomnia is always addressed. Sometimes it is pain or another physical problem. It may be that inactivity and frequent daytime naps make sleep harder to come by at night. If so, a change to the daily routine may be a more satisfactory alternative to sedation. If there are clear signs of emotional distress, allowing the person to talk will be an important and necessary part of the care. There is also a well known yoga technique that can, at times, be of benefit. It involves focussing on the in and out breaths and the movement of the abdomen during the breathing cycle. This 'mild' meditative practice often settles a racing mind and the endless cycle of thoughts that prevent sleep.

Sedation has a limited role but may be used for brief periods to re-establish a normal sleep pattern if this has been disturbed by hospitalisation or an altered home environment. If night sedation is used, do remember:

- Morning drowsiness is a potential problem, particularly if sedation is given later than the recommended time.

- The risk of a fall or other accidents increases with the degree of drowsiness.
- The elderly and frail are more at risk of excessive sedation and so the dose may need to be adjusted.
- A previous history of sedative or heavy alcohol use may render the prescribed sedation less effective.
- Sedation loses its effect over time so is best used for brief periods only.
- Sedation may occasionally cause or contribute to the onset of confusion.
- If reasonable doses of sedation do not achieve the desired effect, consider the possibility of underlying emotional or physical problems.

How do I deal with emergencies?

The likelihood of an emergency is generally small, but being prepared is always a good thing. The most frequently encountered emergencies are listed below. This book provides basic information on most of them, but strategies to prevent and manage those relevant to your loved one's condition should be discussed with the treating doctor. In other words, formulate a plan that is relevant to yours and your loved one's circumstances. Once a plan has been agreed upon, document it and make sure it is kept in a prominent place and that all key people know about it. Ensure you have all the medication and equipment that may be required. Check that you have the phone numbers of people you may need to call. Record business, after-hour and mobile phone numbers and keep these in a very visible spot (e.g. on the fridge door or by the phone).

Emergencies that may require forward planning include:

- pain that does not respond to breakthrough medication
- severe breathlessness
- loss of consciousness

- sudden death
- fitting
- haemorrhage (bleeding)
- confusion
- blocked urinary catheter
- profuse or persistent vomiting
- progressive or sudden weakness and numbness of the legs
- falls

Chapter 5

Day-to-day care

But the pauses between the notes –
ah, there is where the art resides.

ARTUR SCHNABEL

Chapter 5

Day-to-day care

This chapter deals with many of the practical problems encountered in the daily care of a person who is dying. It does not delve into medical or treatment-related issues, as these are covered in other chapters. Instead, it focuses on the basic necessities of life such as food, drink and comfort and how these are provided at the various stages of illness, particularly around the time of death (in palliative circles this form of care is called *supportive care*). Finally, it looks at the quality of human contact and how best to nurture and preserve the dignity of the person who is dying. The comments and observations are made with cancer in mind but most apply in varying degrees to other life-threatening illnesses.

The importance of supportive care hardly needs to be emphasised. From the moment your loved one receives a life-t hreatening diagnosis, you will expend extraordinary amounts of time and energy attempting to sustain their body and nurture their spirit. When medical treatment fails and is ultimately withdrawn, the basic human necessities – food, fluids and comfort – assume even greater significance, as they alone are seen to stand between life and death. Food and fluids, once consumed for sustenance and pleasure, now take on alchemical properties as, together with comfort measures, they become nature's only medicine when death is near.

The value attached to food and fluids can vary enormously with members of the one family, and these differences can cause problems. Some see the dwindling intake as part of the dying process and, while saddened, they accept the inevitability of death. Others are not so prepared to make the shift and may insist on special diets, vitamins or some form of artificial feeding in the belief (hope) that these will relieve suffering and change the course of events. If differences exist, repercussions may be considerable and long-lasting unless resolved early in the course of events.

If the dying person has given some form of advance care directive, all management decisions should be in accordance with that directive. If no such directive exists and the dying person does not or cannot express their wish, a family conference with the treating doctor may resolve any impasse. In most instances, family differences, whether over food, fluids or medications, can be bridged through good communication. An honest appraisal of the situation, the relative merits of treatment and supportive measures will assist in the process. This type of information, given compassionately and clearly, usually forms the basis of a successful resolution.

The need to feed or hydrate someone who is dying often stems from deep-seated grief. This grief often finds an outlet in 'trying to make things better'. If these efforts are misdirected or futile they are not only burdensome to the dying person but also exacerbate the carer's grief. The information that follows will, I hope, go some way to clearing up misconceptions about food, fluids and other forms of supportive care and allow carers to focus on what is possible.

Cancer cures

When someone is told they have cancer, they and their family frequently go in search of treatments that may increase the chance of survival. This is a normal and healthy response but can sometimes get out of hand, consuming the life and time of many people in the process. I am not only referring to complementary and alternative therapies but also to conventional medical treatment.

Considerable uncertainty may exist about the value of medical treatment, particularly chemotherapy and radiotherapy. The benefits they offer are often accompanied by side effects that are as unpleasant as they are unwanted. Despite this, most people with cancer will endure the physical and psychological hardship associated with either or both in the hope that the end will justify the means. Their life can become an endless series of doctor's appointments, clinic visits and tests, but they subject themselves to these and all forms of treatment in the hope of preserving life.

The situation with complementary medicine and alternative therapies is not much different. The range on offer is enormous and continues to increase at a rapid rate. People will try almost anything. Many with cancer will, at some stage of their illness, experiment with a form of complementary therapy and evidence indicates more money is spent on this form of treatment than on chemotherapy. When there is so much at stake, who can blame a person for trying? From the patient's point of view there is much to gain and nothing to lose, even if the medical profession sees it differently.

Sadly, diets, vitamin supplements and purported cancer cures have had little if any impact on the outcome of cancer. We could of course say much the same for chemotherapy, although there have been some spectacular remissions and cures attributed to modern chemotherapy regimes – the American cyclist Lance Armstrong being the classic example. Despite the lack of evidence, we must be careful not to judge those who go in search of cures, but try to understand why they do it. People use complementary medicines and alternative treatments just as they use chemotherapy. Not as a last-ditch measure, but as an opportunity to take some control over their destiny, rather than submit passively to an illness that threatens their existence. It becomes a visible and tangible way of expressing their desire to live and determination not to submit without a fight.

If complementary treatment fails, we must avoid automatically labelling it as a failure and the person's efforts in vain. The example of Judy in Chapter 11, 'The inner journey', shows that any treatment, medical or complementary, cannot be judged only on whether it is successful: it should be judged on what it has meant to the person and how it has influenced their life's journey. I am supportive of people who wish to try complementary medicines or alternative therapies providing:

- there has been a considered decision and not a reflex response to something heard, seen or read about in the media
- it is what the dying person wants rather than what a family member or friend recommends
- it is done at an appropriate time in the illness and not at the eleventh hour
- it does not consume too much valuable time or involve unreasonable travel
- it is within their budget
- it is not unpleasant, dangerous or clearly fraudulent
- it does not interfere with standard treatments
- it does not involve too great a change to the way of life or interfere with pleasurable activities, including the consumption of favourite foods or drinks
- a time is set down to review the treatment and decide whether it should be continued.

Rather than summarise information on the numerous complementary and alternative treatments available I would direct anyone interested in this topic to the National Center [sic] for Complementary and Alternative Medicine (NCCAM) website. The NCCAM is funded by the National Institute of Health in the USA and provides objective and unbiased information on most if not all complementary medicines and alternative treatments currently in use. Its website is as follows: www.nccam.nih.gov/health.

Loss of appetite

Loss of appetite (anorexia) goes hand in hand with advanced (metastatic) cancer, and occurs not infrequently with other serious illnesses. The weight loss that accompanies this symptom is a stark reminder of the underlying illness and its devastating effects. Be aware, however, that there are other causes of anorexia and weight loss. The list is long but chemotherapy, radiotherapy and other medications deserve special mention. More will be said about these later in this chapter.

Once treatable causes have been excluded, numerous medical and proprietary medications are available that may stimulate appetite. Cortisone derivatives (usually dexamethasone) or a hormonal agent called megestrol are perhaps the best of a bad lot. Cortisone is the more popular, but like megestrol the benefits are often temporary and side effects are relatively common.

Weight loss

The body is like any machine – it needs fuel to operate. This fuel comes in the form of food and fluids which supply calories for the body to burn, just as a motor burns petrol. The number of calories we need each day to maintain normal weight and function depends on our age, metabolism and level of activity. What may be sufficient for an elderly, inactive individual would be grossly inadequate for an active teenager in the middle of a growth spurt.

If we exceed our daily caloric needs we put on weight and if this continues unabated we risk becoming obese. If the caloric intake is inadequate, weight loss follows. Starvation is the extreme form of weight loss. Outside of war torn and developing countries we hardly see it today. Cancer, other wasting diseases and anorexia nervosa are, however, the notable causes of extreme weight loss in our Western world.

Like the motor car, the body has its own fuel tank where energy is stored and made available to meet the needs of the body's metabolism.

If fuel (calories) is in short supply and the level in the tank drops, the body adapts by slowing its metabolism, thereby reducing the need for fuel. If this strategy is inadequate and the fuel tank runs dry, energy is obtained from fat stores within the body, which function as a reserve tank. If the shortage continues for a prolonged period, body fat and then muscle will gradually disappear and the person will become thinner, weaker and ultimately wasted – a state of health commonly referred to as *cachexia*.

When weight loss is due to an inadequate intake of calories, as is the case with starvation, feeding, either naturally or artificially via the intravenous or naso-gastric route, provides an immediate source of energy for the body to heal itself. Weight loss ceases, fat stores are replenished, physical strength returns, the fuel tank is topped up and the person starts to look and feel better.

In the context of palliative care, poor appetite and weight loss may be due to any number of factors other than the underlying disease – it can be caused by medication, chemotherapy, radiotherapy, surgery, difficulty swallowing, peptic ulcers, infection or depression. If these respond to appropriate management, appetite usually improves and weight loss is reversed. In the absence of any complicating factors, weight loss is usually related to the disease itself and will continue unless the disease responds to treatment.

When weight loss occurs because of starvation, the body attempts to minimise the loss by slowing the metabolic rate. With cancer the metabolic rate is high and remains high even when food intake is diminished or absent altogether. The reason for this aberration is complex but can be simplified as follows. Cancer is essentially a parasite, living on and deriving energy from its host (the patient). It continues to grow irrespective of how much or how little the person eats, for its growth is independent of the mechanisms that control normal body functions. Even when there is a shortage of calories, cancer cells grow and continue to draw energy from their host, even while the host is losing weight. The greater the number of cancer cells (i.e. the bigger the cancer), the greater the weight loss. It is the cancer's relentless growth and 'thirst' for calories that keep the metabolic rate high and results in the dramatic weight loss we see in people who have advanced cancer (see the table below).

Giving food to those whose weight loss is due to starvation quickly reverses the problem. Unfortunately, the same is not true of cancer. Food will not reverse this weight loss because it feeds the cancer more than it feeds the ailing body – cancer's metabolic rate is so high, it consumes most of the calories while normal tissues miss out. This does not mean you should withhold food from someone with cancer, but food should be given only when the person feels like eating. Feeding someone who has advanced cancer when they are not hungry does not make them feel better, nor does it result in any weight gain. The same is true of anyone with a life-threatening illness irrespective of the cause. The body has its own natural intelligence and will say when it wants food and what type of food it wants or needs.

Loss of appetite with cancer makes some sense and can be seen as the body's way (futile as it may be) of dealing with the problem. It is as if the body recognises its dilemma and switches off its appetite in a desperate attempt to rid itself of the cancer. The opposite also applies, for when the person feels like eating, chances are that food taken at that time may benefit the body more than the cancer.

TABLE 5.1: Changes associated with weight loss due to starvation and cancer

	STARVATION	CANCER
Sensation of hunger	Yes (in early stages)	No
Metabolic rate	Decreased	Increased
Energy source	Fat	Fat and muscle
Effect of eating	Reverses weight loss	Weight loss continues
Effect of IV feeding	Beneficial	Counterproductive

All this has important implications for cancer patients and the way their weight loss is treated. Similarly, the decision for or against intravenous or other artificial means of feeding depends very much on the cause of the problem. The closer someone is to death, the more likely the poor appetite and weight loss is due to the cancer itself and not some other cause. It is therefore most unlikely to respond to any form of artificial feeding.

Food

Most, but not all who are dying, particularly those with cancer, will lose their appetite at some stage. A time will come when the very sight or smell of food may induce nausea. If this happens, it is better to let the dying person dictate what and when they wish to eat, and in what amounts. This is often harder than it sounds as the preparation and presentation of food is another way of showing your love and care, and to stop this seems unnatural and feels wrong. Meals and meal times are more than occasions to eat. They are times of sharing. They are part of the fabric of life. Dispensing with these established routines and traditions can be very painful. Your loved one's dying involves letting go of many things and, for some, food will be one of the losses.

Learning to live is learning to let go.

SOGYAL RIMPOCHE
The Tibetan Book of Living and Dying

Diets of any form (including that for diabetes), health foods and vitamin supplements have by this time outlived their usefulness and should be abandoned unless your relative/friend determines otherwise. Hanging on to these vestiges of treatment often says something about a person's emotional needs, and may require more attention than the weight loss.

The ritual of three meals a day, while natural for healthy people, is totally inappropriate for those with advanced cancer or other life-threatening illnesses. Feeding should be determined by the wishes of the patient, not the time of day. Servings should be small and presented on small plates as the sight of a large amount of food can destroy whatever appetite remains. Allow the person to feed themselves if possible. They value this independence and it gives them control over how much food they want and the speed at which they wish to eat. It may upset you to see how little they consume, but don't be tempted to suggest they eat a little more. If you say this or attempt to feed them that little bit extra, they may take it, not because they want it but only to please you. Remember, their appetite is almost non-existent and what appears a mere morsel to you may be more than enough to satisfy their needs.

> *Angela was an elderly woman dying of cancer. She was cared for by a loving extended family in her own home. Vomiting had been a major ongoing problem for which no cause could be found and all medications had been ineffective in relieving the problem. During one of my visits I noticed Angela was being fed a large meal that would have satisfied the heartiest of appetites. Angela's appetite was almost non-existent but she ate to please her family, who believed feeding was essential for her well-being.*
>
> *When asked, Angela said her appetite had all but gone and the very sight of food often made her sick. Hearing this, the family agreed to give her only what she wanted and when she wanted it. The vomiting stopped and, although her health continued to deteriorate, everyone was grateful this most distressing symptom had settled.*

Certain foods seem to be more popular than others. Ice cream, yoghurt, custard, jelly (in fact, most sweets), smoothies, soups and small sandwiches (without the crust) are frequently eaten while 'mains' are rejected. Tastes do differ, so ask your relative/friend what they would like and make sure you have ample supplies of their preferred option(s). Given the situation, the various nutritional supplements available through chemist shops have no advantage over smoothies or their like.

Thirst is often a greater concern than hunger, so do not be surprised if the desire for fluid outweighs the desire for food. The rule of thumb is to give whatever liquids the person wants, in the amount they choose. Chilled or iced water is most refreshing, but soft drinks, cordials and fruit drinks are frequently requested and provide some variety. Small amounts of alcohol are permitted.

As the illness progresses, the dying person becomes increasingly weak and swallowing more an ordeal. Appetite has by this time all but disappeared. When your loved one is unable to swallow or if they refuse food, concentrate on overall comfort. This includes keeping the mouth moist with small amounts of water or ice (further information follows). Be reassured your relative or friend will not feel hungry and will not die of hunger. They are dying as a result of the illness, and the inability to eat and drink at this late stage is part of the dying process. Do not be side-tracked into doing something about their eating when it is their dying that demands your full attention. They need you more than they need food.

Just as there is no place for food at this stage of a person's life, there is also no role for intravenous fluids. Intravenous fluids have negligible caloric or nutritional value and do not make the dying person feel better; nor do they result in them living longer. Intravenous fluids may in fact make things worse. (I will say more about this later.)

It is okay for you to drink or eat small amounts while in the room, but save larger meals for another time and place. The sight and smell of a cooked meal may not be the best thing for someone already nauseated. If, on the other hand, the person asks you to sit and eat your meal with them, do so as this may indicate a desire to talk.

Fluids

While hunger is rarely a problem in those who are dying, the same cannot be said of thirst. The desire for liquids to quench thirst or soothe a parched throat is a constant issue. Thirst rarely influences the timing of death but it can certainly impair quality of life. The relief of thirst is one of the body's most basic needs and is present throughout life, from birth to death. Fluids are so vital to life that the body has many in-built warning mechanisms to let it know if 'fluid levels' are low. Thirst happens to be one of the very early warning signals. Initially, its message is gentle but if it goes unheard, thirst increases and can become unpleasant. The most common causes of thirst in the palliative care situation are as follows:

- **Inadequate fluid intake.** This is the most obvious and frequently the most common cause. The average daily requirement for a healthy person is 1500–2000 mls/day (equivalent to 6–8 cups), but is in the order of 800–1000 mls/day in those nearing the end of life. Keeping up with this reduced intake can be difficult, particularly if the person depends on others for help.
- **Increased fluid requirements.** Fluid requirements may be greater than normal because of the following:
  - a hot day
  - sweating – a relatively common problem in those with advanced cancer, resulting in increased fluid loss
  - fever and infection
  - vomiting, diarrhoea or fluid loss from any cause
  - medications – for example, tablets used to treat leg oedema (diuretics).
- **Dry mouth.** Causes include:
  - mouth infections, particularly thrush
  - morphine and other analgesics, irrespective of whether they are given by mouth or injection
  - other drugs
  - oxygen, if given without a humidifier.

When trying to prevent or alleviate thirst, always remember to look for causes that may be reversible. Failing that, some practical and useful pointers for dealing with thirst are as follows:

- Although tasteless, water is the best liquid for relieving or preventing thirst, so always keep a supply of cool water within reach.
- Because water is tasteless it is not unusual for someone to 'thirst' for another taste experience; be alert to this and don't be afraid to offer a new taste sensation. Recently, a patient of mine took to lime drinks, having never tried them before.
- We are creatures of habit, so if tea and coffee have been the preferred drinks in health they may be sought after and appreciated in times of illness. Remember, however, tastes can change.
- Alcohol in moderation is fine but it is a mild diuretic, so it may be good for the palate but not so good for alleviating thirst.
- Cool rather than warm/hot fluids are more soothing for a dry or inflamed throat.
- As with food, a small amount of fluid at frequent intervals is better tolerated than a larger volume all at once.
- Some people like to suck ice. Try ordinary ice or small ice-blocks made with Coca-Cola (often recommended by palliative care nurses), other soft drinks, cordials and fruit drinks. This is a tasty and less clinical way of supplementing fluids.
- Drinking through a straw or off a spoon may be easier for those too weak to hold a glass.

Intravenous and subcutaneous infusions

As a person becomes weaker, drowsier and less able to drink, fluid intake is reduced and the problems of dry mouth and thirst increase accordingly. At this point, you may wonder about the place of an intravenous infusion to replace fluids and prevent thirst and dehydration.

For those not familiar with the technology, an intravenous infusion involves the insertion of a cannula (thin plastic tube) into a vein and running saline (salt) or dextrose (sugar) solutions through it to replace fluids or prevent dehydration. More recently, it has been found that inserting a cannula into the tissues directly beneath the skin and running fluids into this space (subcutaneous infusion) is technically easier and equally effective. Unlike the intravenous route, antibiotics, vitamins and many drugs cannot bc administered via this subcutaneous route.

So what is the place of a subcutaneous or intravenous infusion (from here, referred to simply as a 'drip') in people who are too weak or drowsy to swallow? In this situation thirst can only get worse and common sense suggests that a drip is essential. While this is true for someone who has a reversible problem, it is not the case for those approaching death. Let me elaborate.

What symptoms other than thirst occur with dehydration?

Dehydration is a clinical term used when someone is 'dry' or short on fluids. Thirst is the most common and earliest symptom and is the body's prompt to drink more. If the call to quench thirst is not heeded, other symptoms such as weakness, poor concentration, lethargy and confusion may follow. These very same symptoms, however, also result from severe illness so, when present, we cannot automatically assume that dehydration alone is the cause.

Will a drip ease thirst in someone unable to drink?

The only way thirst can be eased is by drinking or by moistening the mouth and lips. No amount of intravenous or subcutaneous fluids will relieve thirst. If a drip is used, intensive mouth care is still mandatory (information on this is provided later in the chapter).

Will a drip prolong life?

If the illness is so advanced as to interfere with swallowing or drinking, death is more likely to result from the illness than the lack of fluids. A drip will not prolong life in this situation.

Will a drip make a dying person feel any better?

No. Most if not all the symptoms (thirst excluded) are due to the illness and will not improve with a drip.

Can a drip make matters worse?

It may not make things worse but a drip can introduce several new problems that complicate care. These problems include frequent urination, which in some instances creates a need for a catheter. Fluid may also accumulate under the skin (oedema), increasing the risk of pressure areas. It may also accumulate in the lungs, leading to 'moist or rattly' breathing and chest infections.

Conclusion

Given these facts, a drip is rarely if ever used in those who are dying. It does not prolong life or relieve thirst and can introduce new and troublesome symptoms.

How to relieve thirst

As already mentioned, the best and easiest way to alleviate thirst in someone who is unable to drink is to keep the mouth and tongue moist. If the person is awake and strong enough to swallow, small amounts of fluids can be given via a straw or by spoon. Small chips of ice to suck are a useful and soothing way to supplement fluids. The resulting fluid intake is relatively small and falls far short of daily requirements but should be enough to keep the mouth moist and relieve thirst. Remember, the goal is not to achieve full fluid replacement, but to give enough liquid to ease thirst.

If a person is unconscious and unable to swallow, the mouth can be kept moist by using artificial saliva sprays or by injecting a small volume of water (1–2 ml) into the mouth via a syringe every hour or thereabouts. This fluid is run in slowly, onto the tongue or between the inside of the bottom lip and the lower gum. This volume, administered regularly (every 30–60 minutes during the day and less frequently at night), is large enough to keep the mouth moist and small enough to be absorbed without the need to swallow. If necessary, a nurse can also show you how to clean the mouth and keep it moist by using damp swabs. This can be done in combination with any or all of the above measures.

Drips are rarely if ever indicated. If they are used it is often to appease a relative's grief rather than the dying person's needs. Some family members cannot cope with the thought of their loved one not drinking and will request a drip. Others may ask because of their cultural, religious or spiritual beliefs. Whatever the reason, palliative care respects all reasonable requests. Let me illustrate with the following two examples.

Joseph had been admitted to the hospice for the relief of pain associated with cancer of the liver. The cancer was far advanced and, although the pain was quickly controlled, Joseph's condition deteriorated rapidly. He was dying and both he and his family were informed of this at a bedside meeting. In the space of one week Joseph became increasingly drowsy and ultimately unconscious. As he was unable to swallow, mouth care was commenced and pain relief continued. Joseph appeared to be very comfortable.

His wife was distraught and initially I attributed this to grief about her husband's impending death, but as we spoke it became clear there was more to her distress. Both she and Joseph had strong spiritual values that included a belief in reincarnation. They believed that to die in a state of 'dehydration' would seriously compromise the reincarnation process. She wondered if there was something that could be done. Putting my medical prejudice aside, I mentioned an infusion which she readily and happily embraced. Joseph died two days after a subcutaneous infusion had been commenced and his wife, though grieving, was much more at peace about the way he died.

Tsung was an elderly Chinese woman, dying from cancer of the stomach. She had been cared for at home by a large and loving family until she fell and broke her hip. Severe pain necessitated admission to the hospice and an increased dose of morphine. Her condition deteriorated and, while the family could accept the inevitability of her death, they wished to demonstrate their love and respect for all she had done by continuing to offer her sustenance. They asked that we not only start an infusion but that vitamins be added to the infusion to ensure she was not vitamin-deficient. It made no medical sense but it was culturally and personally important to the family that this should be done. Accordingly, an intravenous infusion containing vitamins was commenced and continued to the time of her death several days later.

Bowel care

You may have noticed that in caring for someone who is unwell a lot of emphasis is placed on the 'bowels'. Constipation can be a very real and painful problem for anyone, particularly those who are weak and bed-bound. Chronic ill health, altered eating habits, reduced food and fluid intake and inactivity combine to make constipation a common problem among palliative care patients.

Surprisingly, a regular bowel motion is just as normal for someone who is unwell and eats little (or nothing at all) as it is for those who are healthy. The reason is that the bulk of a bowel motion comes from two sources—the residue of what we eat and the natural shedding of cells that line the full length of the bowel (6-8 metres). These cells are shed and renewed on a daily basis and, given the length of the bowel and the number of cells involved, their contribution to the size of a bowel motion is substantial.

There is no precise definition for constipation and what one person may label 'constipation' another may not. So constipation is relative, but can be said to exist if someone's bowels do not open as often as is normal for them, or if the act of trying to pass a bowel motion is painful, or if after passing a motion a feeling of incomplete emptying remains. The belief that someone's bowels should open every day is therefore erroneous but anything less than three times a week may be a problem.

The chances of constipation are extremely high in the palliative care population, not only for the reasons mentioned above but also because of the effects of morphine. Morphine and most pain relievers are constipating, so preventive measures are almost always necessary. There is no strong pain reliever that does not cause constipation and so it is always going to be a problem if pain relief is required. Morphine and preparations containing codeine, such as Panadeine Forte®, are probably the worst offenders. Morphine has a particularly bad reputation for causing constipation – I liken it to cement, as it can cause the bowel motion to set like concrete if it is 'left too long'. Some of the newer analgesics are not as constipating and can be used or substituted if constipation is obstinate.

Any ill person whose lifestyle and eating habits have altered is at risk of constipation and may benefit from preventive measures. Unfortunately, many of the recommendations given to 'healthy' people (e.g. increased intake of fluids and dietary fibre, and increased activity) may be difficult if not impossible to implement in those who are unwell. Friends and health care professionals all have their favourite recipes. I regularly recommend kiwi fruit (one or more per day), prunes and Bekunis® (senna) tea. If these and other simple measures fail to prevent constipation your loved one may (will, if morphine is on their list of medications) need laxatives.

The range of laxatives is enormous, suggesting there is no single outstanding or universally acceptable agent. To make matters worse, most are fairly mild and the number of tablets or the volume of liquid required to do the job (excuse the pun) often reaches prohibitive proportions. Laxatives are not free of side effects and must always be used in the recommended dose. The most frequently prescribed laxatives are Coloxyl® tablets, with or without senna, and Movicol®. Actilax®, Duphalac® and Sorbilax® are also used, but some find these preparations too sweet and nauseating. Their laxative action also depends on a good intake of fluid (at least 1000–1500 ml/day), and this may not be possible with someone who is ill.

One would think a diagnosis of constipation is easy to make, but it remains one of the most frequently overlooked problems in those who are sick and dying. Apart from the obvious discomfort, constipation can cause pain in the lower abdomen, nausea, vomiting, difficulty in passing urine (yes, urine) and very occasionally restlessness and confusion. So keep a record of when the bowels open and tell the doctor or nurse if they have not worked for several days. They will make their own assessment, which generally involves a few questions, a feel of the abdomen and, occasionally, an x-ray of the abdomen and an internal examination through the anus. The latter is not painful but is often described as uncomfortable and undignified. It is not done routinely, only when there is some doubt about the diagnosis.

If constipation is confirmed, a larger than usual dose of Movicol, suppositories or an enema are commonly used to rectify the problem. It might seem heavy handed resorting to such measures in those who are sick or dying but, conscious or not, people still feel discomfort from constipation, and not uncommonly they can become restless and agitated. Appropriate treatment of the constipation is often required for these people to settle. So, if ever your dying relative becomes restless or agitated, do not be surprised if the doctor or nurse raises the possibility of constipation or a full bladder (see below).

Bladder care

Difficulty or an inability to pass urine (the latter is called *urinary retention*) is a relatively frequent occurrence in those (especially men) who are confined to bed. Urinary retention can result in severe abdominal pain and generally requires some form of intervention such as a catheter. The problem, however, is frequently overlooked for the following reason. It is not unusual for someone with urinary retention to pass (dribble) small amounts of urine and this often diverts attention away from the possibility of a blockage. In reality, this is an overflow situation and the key symptoms are worsening abdominal pain, an inability to pass urine or the ability to pass only a few drops at a time. If any of these problems occur, always report them to the palliative care team as early as possible.

If a catheter is required it can, in most instances, be inserted at home. If there is a high risk of urinary retention, a urinary catheter may be recommended as a precautionary measure. There are benefits, but also drawbacks to doing this so the decision always entails appropriate discussion with patient and family.

A catheter is inserted via the penis in men and the urethra in women; in both instances this is referred to as a *urethral catheter*. Local anaesthetic renders the procedure relatively pain-free and the relief that follows quickly atones for any discomfort associated with the catheter's insertion. Much less frequently, the catheter will be inserted through the lower abdomen. This is called a *supra-pubic catheter* and is indicated if previous attempts at inserting a urethral catheter have been difficult or when a catheter is required for a long period of time. Urethral catheters are changed every 4 to 6 weeks. They, like supra-pubic catheters, increase the risk of a urinary infection, which usually manifests as cloudy or smelly urine, a fever or confusion (especially in the elderly).

When a person is drowsy or too weak to use a toilet or bedpan, the most common scenario is urinary incontinence. Inability to control the flow of urine can result in the embarrassment of a wet bed. The inability to control one's bladder and bowels is one of the biggest concerns most people have when dying. They may accept or resign themselves to the fact they are dying, but the loss of control over vital functions is another matter. Knowing someone else will have to attend to them (and a soiled or wet bed) is a constant source of worry and embarrassment. I have no simple solution, but if I were the patient I would find the following words (or something similar) comforting: 'We love you, and while we know you are embarrassed, we want to care for you even if that means wiping your bottom and changing a wet bed'. Knowing my family can do it, and choose to do it, would go a long way towards easing my concern.

There are many aids to help with urinary incontinence. A urethral catheter is one, but there are alternatives. Most of the alternatives are available for use at home (as well as in the hospice/hospital) and can be obtained through the community or palliative care nurses. The nurses are the best people to advise you on all aspects of bladder care, so take time to talk to them even if there is no problem. It is better to be prepared.

You might think that urine output should diminish and wet beds would be rare with someone who drinks very little. Prepare yourself for a surprise. People continue to pass reasonable amounts of urine for quite some time after they stop drinking. This is because the body is like a sponge and contains an extraordinary amount of water even in those with a poor fluid intake. Apart from causing embarrassment, wet beds are unpleasant and uncomfortable, irritate the skin and increase the risk of skin breakdown and pressure areas. While prevention may not always be possible, a prompt change of bed linen and pyjamas helps preserve skin integrity and an individual's dignity.

We are conditioned not to wet the bed so a full bladder is one of many things that can wake a person, sick or healthy, from sleep. If the person is deeply unconscious, they may not wake but become restless and start to groan. Restlessness in someone previously comfortable or asleep suggests some form of discomfort or pain. A full bladder and a wet bed are two of the many possibilities. So, rather than reach for a booster dose of morphine or extra sedation, look for a cause and if you do not find one and the restlessness persists, seek professional help.

Skin care and pressure areas

As a person's health deteriorates the amount of time spent in bed or a chair increases dramatically and, for someone who has lost weight, these natural and seemingly innocuous positions can present special problems. The fragility of the skin, loss of skin elasticity and tissue padding make weight-bearing areas particularly susceptible to damage. The problem is compounded by weakness that may limit a person's ability to change position and relieve pressure. So when someone is ill and confined to bed or chair, the skin over weight-bearing areas such as buttocks, sacrum, hips, heels and elbows is prone to damage. The result can be a loss of normal skin integrity, leading to tears or ulcers, both of which are called pressure areas. These pressure areas may be small or large and are often painful and debilitating. They are prone to infection, which results in more pain and significantly delays healing.

The earliest warning sign of a pressure area is redness in one or more of the sites mentioned above. If you notice this, tell the community nurse or doctor immediately. The earlier the problem is treated the more likely it will heal with less pain and fewer complications. In the earliest stages, treatment may involve repositioning, but dressings and sometimes pain relief are necessary once the skin is broken. The dressings are usually done by the community nurses. The frequency of the dressings depends on the site and size of the damaged skin. The nurses will also show you how best to reposition your loved one. These positions are often hard to maintain. They are less comfortable than lying on one's back and often compromise a person's independence. How strictly you enforce the repositioning does therefore depend on circumstances. The overall comfort of the person in the bed should always take precedence.

Prevention is, of course, better than cure and I recommend you speak to the nurses about how to maintain skin integrity. Depending on the circumstances, pressure areas may be difficult or near impossible to prevent and may appear despite the best care. So do not blame yourself if one or more appear. The following precautionary measures may, however, help:

- the correct choice of bedding, mattress and chair (the nurse or occupational therapist can advise on this)
- correct undercover for sacrum and heels (e.g. sheepskin rug, boots)
- regular change of position
- keeping susceptible areas clean and dry

- careful application of appropriate creams as recommended by chemist or nurse
- changing a wet or moist bed and pyjamas as soon as either is noted.

Mouth care

The problems of thirst and dry mouth have been discussed earlier in this chapter under the headings of 'Fluids' and 'How to relieve thirst'.

Oral thrush (also called *monilia* or *candidiasis*) is one of the most overlooked infections in the sick and dying. It may be encountered at any time in the course of an illness, but is much more common in the later stages. Thrush is a fungal infection. It appears as white plaques inside the mouth and is most commonly seen on the roof of the mouth. It is easily missed so careful inspection with a good torch is required if you suspect thrush. It is more common in those who have been or are still taking antibiotics or cortisone (dexamethasone, prednisolone and prednisone). Thrush causes few early symptoms but left untreated will result in a sore throat and difficulty with swallowing. I have seen many people who were unable to swallow food or fluids simply because of thrush.

Many agents can be used to treat this condition but the most popular are nystatin (Nilstat® or Mycostatin®) drops. The drops may sting a little when first used but this is due to the underlying inflammation and not the drops. The drops should be swished around the mouth and kept there as long as possible before they are swallowed or spat out. The drops are yellow in colour and often stain the tongue. This is nothing to worry about. As thrush is often present under dentures it is important to give these a good soak in bicarbonate solution at least once a day. If the thrush is stubborn it may be advisable to leave the dentures out for a good part of the day and at night or, if preferred, for one hour after the drops have been installed.

Bicarbonate mouthwashes are routinely recommended (four times daily) to prevent thrush in susceptible patients. It is better not to swallow the mouthwash, but no harm results if this happens inadvertently. The mouthwash is made by adding half a teaspoon of bicarbonate to a 250mls (one cup) of water. The solution can also be used to soak dentures. More potent antifungal medication is available for the more severe forms of thrush or for those who do not respond to the usual local treatment(s).

Other infections are far less common, but I will mention mouth ulcers and gingivitis because they, too, are painful. Like thrush, they can be difficult to diagnose, so ask your doctor to review the situation if your loved one complains of a persistent sore throat or mouth. Very rarely, a mumps-like infection can occur when the salivary glands in front of the ears swell and become painful. This is not mumps but results in symptoms and signs very similar to that once common childhood infection. It is due to a bacterial infection (mumps is due to a virus) and settles with antibiotics and good mouth care.

As health deteriorates and fluid intake is reduced, a person may find it increasingly difficult to swallow tablets and it is not unusual to discover them untouched on the bedside table or partly dissolved in the mouth. If this is the case, you can ask the doctor to review the medication, as all except those given for pain and symptom relief can now be ceased. Those that are essential can usually be given by another route – for example, injection under the skin (subcutaneous) – thereby reducing the tablet burden without compromising pain or symptom control.

The final word on mouth care concerns dentures, which by this time are usually ill fitting and may be more of a nuisance than an asset. The decision to leave them in or out is obviously up to the individual, and appearances as much as comfort will influence the ultimate choice. If your relative is concerned about appearances, he/she may be happy to leave them out most of the time and replace them only when visitors arrive.

Wound care

Open wounds, skin ulceration and pressure areas should be inspected daily, kept clean and dry and covered with a protective dressing. Exposing simple wounds to direct sunlight for one or more hours a day can be beneficial but is of questionable value if the wound is infected or contains unhealthy tissue. It is best to keep these wounds covered, partly for cosmetic reasons, but also to shield the wound from flies.

Holistic care

> *The way care is given can reach the most hidden places.*
>
> DAME CICELY SAUNDERS

The majority of supportive care measures I have described so far relate to physical comfort. While this is important, there are two other important aspects of care. They are a need for purpose or meaning in one's life and the need to maintain relationships. Together these can be viewed as essential CPR for those who are dying, where CPR stands for Comfort, Purpose and Relationships.

These aspects of care are not independent of each other and changes in one can have positive or negative effects on the others. For example, purpose and dignity are often restored when pain is controlled. Similarly, someone may complain of 'pain' when other aspects of their life or relationships are compromised. This interrelationship between body, mind and spirit is well known and the combination of physical pain, mental anguish and existential angst, so often seen in the dying, is usually referred to as *total pain* or *suffering*.

Circumstances determine the relative importance of physical, mental and existential pain but in the context of palliative care it seems that physical pain, when present, overrides all other needs. So one of the goals of palliative care is, whenever possible, to relieve or ease somatic (physical) pain. In so doing, we not only improve comfort and the quality of the person's life but also help restore dignity and purpose, and allow nurturing relationships to resume.

Visits

In the context of ill health, visits are a very important part of social interaction and are often the only avenue a dying person has of maintaining contact with colleagues, friends and even family. Those who are dying frequently lose interest in television, newspapers and local events and, as their world narrows, the only contact between them and the outside is family and friends that visit. Visits are also a way for people to show they care and, ill as their relative/friend may be, the significance of a visit is never lost. People who are dying seek genuine human contact and this genuineness is reflected not only in the frequency of visits, but also in their quality.

Alternatively, it can become a source of concern when a sick person realises that friends have stopped visiting or phoning. Circumstances may play a big part in this, but so often visits and phone calls from friends and colleagues simply dry up. This is often painful and may add to the feeling of alienation that dying people sometimes experience.

Visits can also bring their own problems. Some visitors may stay too long, come more often than seems necessary, say inappropriate things or make unrealistic statements. It is not unreasonable for you, as the carer, to ask people to ring days rather than minutes before they come, not only as a matter of courtesy but also to check whether your loved one is up to taking visitors. Most people will understand if it is not okay or if the visit needs to be cancelled at the last moment. Asking potential visitors to ring also allows you to exert some discretion and to select only those your loved one wants to see. It can be difficult to say no, but if your loved one is too sick or exhausted or wishes not to see certain people, those visits will only add to his/her distress.

If the timing and circumstances are okay, let visitors know how long they can stay, and ask them to keep to that time. Also, suggest they be alert to what is happening – if the sick person looks tired or is dropping off to sleep, or if other visitors arrive, these may be cues to leave earlier rather than later. Most visitors are unsure how long they should stay – guidelines are often gratefully received and could protect you from the embarrassing situation of asking them to leave.

During visits it is not unusual for friends or relatives to ask if there is some way they can help. As a carer you may, for a multitude of reasons, decline this offer. You may feel it is your duty to do everything, you may be embarrassed about accepting help, believe acceptance indicates you are not coping or you may not want 'to put others to the trouble'. Whatever the reason, it is an offer you should not pass up. Not only will it relieve you of some of the more tedious chores, it will free you to spend more quality time with your loved one, family or simply to have time alone. Do not ask too much of yourself or expect that you can take on the task of caring without outside help. We all have our limits and it is better to live within these limits rather than stretch yourself to breaking point. You, your loved one and your family will all benefit from offers of outside help.

With this in mind, have a list of chores that others can do. This is not only liberating for you, it can also be deeply rewarding for others to know they can be of help and that you trust them enough to ask. Tasks may include shopping, cooking a meal once a week, doing the washing, vacuuming the house, mowing lawns, gardening, or spending time with your loved one while you shop, go for a walk or watch a movie. These requests should not be confined only to this time of caring. They are just as helpful and rewarding in the weeks and months following your loved one's death.

Presencing: tips for visitors

To be fully present with someone is not a skill many of us possess. To be present means being fully aware of the moment, hearing what is being said, not looking for answers or solutions to problems, respecting the value of silence and speaking from the heart. Patrick Duignan from the Australian Catholic University defines *presence* as, 'the sacred stillness within the precious space created between people with meaningful relationships'. He goes on to say, 'it is the glue that binds relationships' and quotes the spiritual teacher Eckhart Tolle as saying, 'being present is infinitely more powerful than anything one can say or do...'. Being present not only means you are physically present, but that you are also fully aware of what is happening inside you and around you, and that you respond accordingly.

So, being present is a tall order, but is the mainstay of any relationship and is particularly precious for those who are dying. Visitors who engage in meaningless conversation add to the dying person's suffering. The sick dispense with superficial distractions and focus only on what is truly important. My friend the late Professor Grahame Jones journalled the last few months of his life in his book *Magnanimous Despair*, in which he makes the following plea, 'let the healthy talk of illness, let the sick speak of more important things'.

The biggest concern for people who visit a dying friend or relative is, 'what do I say?' To visit with a pre-planned conversation in mind is counterproductive as this is usually done for our benefit and is unlikely to be of any value for the person we visit. So, as threatening as it may seem, it is best if you enter with a clear mind and an open heart and allow the conversation to flow rather than be controlled. A commonly used palliative care adage is, when visiting patients we should always leave our baggage at the front door. Being fully present is hard work, and so too is being authentic. The following points may help you to be present and authentic:

- Listening is more important than speaking (we have two ears and only one mouth).
- Be aware of how you feel and try not to let this influence your words or actions (the story of Helen that follows will illustrate what this means).

- Your body language will make a greater impression than any of the words you use. So sit rather than stand, near rather than far away, make good eye contact and be fully aware of what is happening with the person you are visiting.
- Be real and authentic. You cannot make your friend/relative better nor should you try. They know if you are playing this game and will go along with it, at their own expense. If you do this it is often because you're uncomfortable and unsure about what to say. Being real and authentic means saying 'I don't know what to say' when that is how you feel.
- Respect silence. A lot is happening during these times so don't destroy the chemistry with anxiety-relieving statements or questions.
- If you say something you wished you hadn't said, say so. Such honesty is liberating and much better than a quick change of subject.
- Avoid false claims such as 'You look so much better' (when they don't). They know when you are being 'nice'.
- People don't change because they are dying and nor should you so, bearing in mind all that has been said, relate to the person as you always have in the past.

The American author and caregiver Ram Dass recounts the following story from one of the workshops conducted by Dr Elisabeth Kübler-Ross, a Swiss-born psychiatrist who lived and practiced in America and who became famous for her pioneering work on death and dying.

Helen was a young woman in her mid-thirties. She was a widow with two children, aged 7 and 9 years. Cancer of the breast had been diagnosed two years earlier and, despite multiple operations, chemotherapy and radiotherapy, the disease had spread to her liver, lungs and bones and she was expected to die in a matter of months. Although very thin and weak she had decided to attend one of Elisabeth Kübler-Ross's workshops.

During this workshop she asked those present how they would feel if they came to visit her. Most said they would feel sadness. Sad that a mother of two children was dying so young, or that she would not see her kids grow up or sad for the children. Others said they would feel anxious about what to say and others would feel angry that someone in her situation should be so afflicted. After a while, Helen said that if any of these people came to visit they would be so weighed down by their own grief they would have little room for her pain. The visit may help them, but it would be of little benefit to her.

The moral of this story, which is particularly pertinent to carers and immediate family, is that it is very hard to be there for someone if you are weighed down by your own grief. 'When we are too full of our own suffering we cannot accept the suffering of others', says Merrill Collett in his book *At Home with Dying*. Not only is it hard to be there, but this form of suffering can also lead you to distance yourself physically and/or emotionally from your loved one at a time when you both need each other. If this situation continues, the resulting distress further compounds each other's grief and the ramifications may spill over to involve other family members as they themselves see what is unfolding. The situation may be resolved by open and honest communication or may require the expertise of a counsellor.

Precious normality

One of the very sad things about dying is that the closer someone is to death the more likely they are to be treated as a patient rather than a person. Treatments, tests, visits to doctors and visits by nurses all add up and rob sick and dying people of normal living. Grahame Jones described what it is like when he said, 'What I detest is how effectively the procedure of the treatment robs me of my precious normality and seriously affects my morale'.

Illness can rob people (patients and relatives) of precious normality and, while you may have little control over this, it is important that you and your loved one do not become victims in the process. Retain as much as you can of what is normal in your life irrespective of what else is happening around you. Not only should you seek to retain what is normal, you should guard it as you would anything of value. There are many obstacles, but the benefits derived from such an investment make it worthwhile for you (the carer) and your family and for the one who is dying.

What is normal and of value for the dying person is something that you as relative, carer or friend would know and can therefore maintain and guard. For some it may be reading and, when that is no longer possible, they may like to be read to. For others it may be listening to music, watching videos, doing crosswords, sitting in a much loved garden, emailing friends, writing poetry, having a few drinks or going to the 'local' once a week.

Most important of all is the maintenance (as much as the illness allows) of the previous patterns of intimacy, sensual and sexual sharing. Illness may weaken the body but the desire for closeness and intimacy is never lost. Do not let illness or the fear of causing pain come between you and the one you love. If the one who is dying is your spouse or partner, whatever the time of day or night, do not be afraid to hop into bed with them, cuddle, caress and be as sensual as circumstances allow. Protect such intimate moments by taking the phone off the hook and putting a 'do not disturb' sign on the front door. Everything else can wait. For all others, closeness is something that must be respected, but not abused. Maintain a level of closeness similar to that which existed before the illness. Anything more or less is not only artificial but also patronising.

For the one who is sick, some of what was normal may no longer be possible. Common sense must prevail. The realisation they can no longer do some of the things they once enjoyed or things that were once part of normal life is painful and confronting. Rather than destroying 'precious normality', such realisations introduce a measure of reality and direct the person to invest more time in things that are not only normal but also possible.

Creating a nurturing physical environment is a useful and meaningful exercise for you to engage in with your loved one as it not only gets priorities in order but can be a healing and cathartic process for both. Here are some peripheral but related things to consider:

- Protect and maintain a normal home environment by censoring any unnecessary or unwanted visits.
- Prepare for dying but not at the expense of living.
- Have the dying person spend most of their day in the place they prefer, doing what they choose (within reason).
- Get full value out of their favourite clothing, CDs or books.
- Maintain your usual routines and habits, while that is possible.
- Keep a regular check on needs and preferences.
- Keep the medical paraphernalia in another room if at all possible.
- Make appropriate adjustments to 'precious normality' depending on your loved one's needs and state of health.

Jessie was resident in a nursing home for six months prior to her death. For all but the last 2 weeks of her life she was active and alert and wanted her room to be a reflection of the family home she had lived in for 40 years. She had a clock on the wall, photos of her family and grandchildren, a TV to watch her favourite programs, a radio to listen to in the dead of night and frequent visits from all the family. It became her home away from home.

Following the first of two strokes, Jessie was unable to speak, but she was clearly afraid and wanted her family to be with her as much as time allowed. A greeting and parting kiss were no longer sufficient. She needed hugs, cuddles and kisses and no amount of contact was too much. A second stroke one week later rendered her unconscious. She did not respond to the spoken word but seemed to rouse whenever she was held. The TV and the hoards of visitors now seemed out of place and the family felt she would at this time in her life want only her immediate family around. A roster was drawn up and from that moment on Jessie was never alone. She died just as she would have wished, surrounded by her mementos and her family.

Caring for the carer

Time is in short supply for the one who is dying and so their wish to make the most of every moment is not unreasonable. This is easier said than done, particularly for the carer. To be 'on call' 24 hours a day and to cater to every wish can be extraordinarily hard, not only because of the physical task but also because of the emotional effort required. Such commitment is often beyond one person's capacity. Be realistic in what you can do and don't be afraid to ask for help. Acknowledge what is going on inside of you and, if necessary, find somebody you can confide in. Frustration, helplessness and anger are not uncommon and are very normal in this situation. You are the primary carer and unless you care for yourself it is very hard to care for someone else, even when that person is one you love dearly.

Your survival depends on you being able to preserve some of your own precious normality, whether that is an afternoon nap, a weekly game of golf or bowls, a morning with friends, shopping or going to the movies. These things should not be regarded as luxuries that you can no longer afford but as essential for preserving your own emotional and physical well-being. They are as essential as regular meals and sleep. Looking after someone who is dying can be compared to running a marathon. The prime goal of any runner is to finish and that is more likely if they pace themselves from the start. As conditions change, the way they run the race will also change. And that is how it should be for you as the carer. Go slowly at the start, adjust your pace depending on the circumstances and aim to be there in one piece at the end of your race.

In the men's marathon at the 1968 Mexico City Olympics, John Stephen Akhwari was the last runner to finish and he entered the stadium one hour after the winner had crossed the line. He was bruised and battered from an earlier fall. Rather than quit he continued running and hobbled exhausted across the finishing line. When asked why he continued running to the finish he said, 'My country did not send me to Mexico City to start the race. They sent me to finish'. This wisdom can be applied to many things in life but no more so than the situation you now find yourself in.

Chapter 6

States of consciousness

To die, to sleep;
To sleep: perchance to dream: ay, there's the rub;
For in that sleep of death what dreams may come,
When we have shuffled off this mortal coil...

WILLIAM SHAKESPEARE
Hamlet, Act III, Scene I

Chapter 6

States of consciousness

As a palliative care doctor for more than twenty years I have been involved in the care of many people who have died. The experience of caring for your loved one may lead you to wonder how anyone could do this type of work. Rest assured you are not the only one who thinks this way. Whenever the topic of work comes up in conversation, as it often does, there is always a pregnant pause after I tell people about my line of work. If it is not their words, it is their body language that gives them away. They are clearly taken aback. If I get the chance to ask what it is about palliative care that makes them uncomfortable, most mention sadness and/or fear. Sadness related to loss of life and fear of the unknown. There is no denying those emotions go with the territory. But what these people and others like them fail to appreciate is that in caring for the dying we get to know them and their family intimately and that the work takes us into the 'deep shadows of mystery and the unknown' (Thomas Moore, *Care of the Soul*).

The mystery is death. Until relatively recent times, death had great religious significance and was considered an almost mystical event, even though it carried with it all the same emotions we feel today. A scientific and secular revolution over the past 100 years has seen this mystical component seriously challenged, with death now reduced to the biological equivalent of an 'amen' – the end to a litany of physiological changes and medical interventions. It is, however, ironic that, as death takes on more of a biological status, extraordinary and unusual things are being increasingly reported at and around this time. These events, such as the near-death experience (NDE), deathbed visions (DBV) and out-of-body experiences (OBE), defy rational explanation and do, in their own way, challenge the contemporary reductionist view of death prevalent today.

This chapter looks at some of these strange and extraordinary events. Many are unique to death and are poorly understood, but each serves to reinforce the sense of mystery that characterises the dying process. Death will always remain a mystery and the goal is not to uncover the mystery or the unknowable, for that is impossible, but to learn as much as we can about the unknown. The more we know about the dying process and the events that accompany it, the more we will come to respect it.

Unconsciousness

One of the mysteries is the so-called unconscious state. This is a state that many of us will go through before we die. We recognise it, and say a person is 'unconsciousness' when they no longer respond to the spoken word and make no purposeful movement. In other words it is defined by a lack of action, but does that mean the mind is not functioning? No one really understands what happens or indeed if anything happens in the mind of someone who is unconscious, but the word suggests there is no consciousness or awareness.

When we talk about states of consciousness, most people are familiar with the two extremes – consciousness and unconsciousness – and naturally believe one is the exact opposite of the other. If we accept consciousness to be a state of awareness in which we assimilate information, process it and respond appropriately, then unconsciousness, by definition, is a state where there is no awareness, no processing of information and an inability to act.

Arnold Mindell in his book *Coma: Key to Awakening* says, 'There are powerful and dramatic events trying to unfold themselves in comatose states and nothing happens in coma that is not trying to happen to people all the time'. Such a comment flies in the face of our conventional understanding of coma (unconsciousness) and, if true, would greatly alter the way we relate to and care for those who are unconscious.

Many of my patients prefer to die at home and Pam was no exception. She had a long history of bowel cancer that had continued to grow despite various forms of chemotherapy. Her appetite waned, she lost a considerable amount of weight and ultimately weakness confined her to bed. There was little pain and only small doses of morphine were required to keep her comfortable. Slowly, the weakness overcame her mind as well as her body and she changed from being someone who loved to read and interact with family and friends to someone who slept most of the time, and then to not waking at all. Pam had become unconscious.

Pam was so deeply unconscious she did not react when the nurses inserted a urethral catheter into her bladder. After several days of not responding, eating or drinking I told the family that death was at hand. I visited the next day and there was no change. The following day I rang to see if Pam was still alive and to my surprise I was told she was not only alive but very much awake. She was eating, drinking champagne and entertaining the family. It was her birthday! Later that day she returned to her bed, fell asleep and died 24 hours later.

Stories such as this are not uncommon and certainly challenge the medical profession's long-held belief that unconsciousness, or coma, is a mindless interlude between life and death. The mystery deepened when I realised that many of the patients that woke (albeit temporarily) had some awareness of events during their period of unconsciousness. Sometimes, this awareness was minimal but others could remember events that family and others had forgotten. In Pam's case it is not unreasonable to suggest her period of wakefulness may have been related to her birthday, and that she had some awareness of this event even though she had been unconscious for several days before.

Angela's story adds to the mystery and, like many of the experiences encountered around death (or near death), it cannot be explained rationally.

Angela was 42 when she died of longstanding cancer. She was the mother of two young children so her death was associated with enormous sadness and grief. As is my practice I visited Angela's family later in the day. Her husband Bill was unsettled and asked me to stay awhile. He then told me of what had happened earlier in the day. Angela's elder sister was terribly upset because of a long-forgotten memory that came flooding back hours after her sister's death. That morning she told Bill how Angela, as a young girl, was very ill from septicaemia and that everyone, including the doctors, had expected her to die. Miraculously, she recovered, but some time after the event Angela told her sister that, as she lay there unconscious, she heard a voice say she would survive the septicaemia but would die at the age of forty two.

Many similar stories suggest that those who are unconscious are not oblivious to what is happening around them and that their level of awareness may be much greater than we have until now considered possible – some have said these people are not unconscious, but superconscious or omniconscious. It also indicates how little we know about death and dying and how much we take for granted. This is particularly true for the medical profession, a profession that devotes so much of its time, effort and money to investigating cures but so little to the understanding and treatment of death and dying, something we shall all one day face. The American physician Eric Krakauer recognised this paradox when he said, 'We as physicians attend to the dying every day but we have not attended to dying itself'.

Awareness during unconsciousness

Awareness during unconsciousness is not just confined to those who are dying. A large study involving 2517 anaesthetised patients, published in 1996 by Drs Philip Merikle and Meredyth Daneman, concluded that information unconsciously perceived during anaesthesia is remembered for many hours. If the information is personally relevant and meaningful, the memory may remain for weeks. This form of remembering is unlike that which operates in our normal waking life. Information perceived during unconsciousness may or may not be remembered, but will still influence how we feel.

As many of the people I care for pass through a stage of unconsciousness before they die, I embarked on a study to see whether awareness could be documented during this time. This seemed important, not only from an academic standpoint, but also because a positive finding could influence our understanding of the dying process and the way care is delivered at this time. During the study we used an instrument that recorded brainwave activity and converted the result to a numerical score that accurately reflected the level of awareness. A score of 100 indicated a fully aware or wide-awake state while zero meant brain death and, obviously, no awareness. To put this in perspective, a level of 50–55 is what anaesthetists aim for during anaesthesia, and with sleep the score can fluctuate between 40 and 80, depending on the stage of sleep.

After the necessary ethical, patient and family approvals process we used this instrument to study the level of awareness in twelve people who were dying (ten with cancer, one with cardiac failure and one with AIDS). The study began the moment each person became unconsciousness and continued until the time of death. The results were surprising, to say the least.

The average score at the time of unconsciousness was 55 and just prior to death it was 44. Both these levels are equivalent to a deeply anaesthetised state and suggest little, if any, possibility of awareness. In all subjects the score was not static but varied depending on circumstances. In many instances it rose to 60–80 with turning or when pain was evident. This left me in no doubt that unconscious patients feel pain and their level of awareness increases to almost wakefulness when pain is present. This was not unexpected and supported the long-held conviction that comfort and ongoing pain relief is essential in those who are unconsciousness. While this came as no surprise, the observation that similar fluctuations in awareness also occurred in the absence of pain was unexpected.

Alberto was the first person we monitored in this study. At the time the machine was connected he was deeply unconscious and unresponsive, even when turned. His reading was 40. No sooner had I connected the machine, than the bedside phone rang and the level immediately jumped to 65, suggesting that the ring had at least registered in his mind. Seeing this, his mother asked whether the same response might occur if she spoke to her son. Not sure of what to expect and fearing disappointment if there was no response, I hesitatingly agreed. She bent over and whispered into his ear. Much to my relief and her joy the reading shot up to 65 and, while no physical changes were noted, the reading remained at that level for the brief time she spoke to him and a little while after.

This increased awareness in response to sound or noise was a reasonably common finding in our study and supports the widely held view that hearing is the last sense to go in those dying and is preserved late into the unconscious period. Even more startling was the occasion when one of the subjects woke from a deeply unconscious state, communicated with her family for approximately 30 minutes and then lapsed back into unconsciousness. I spoke to the family shortly afterwards and they said their mother woke and said goodbye. Interestingly, all the family were present at this time. She died several days later.

There were two other important observations from this study:

- People continue to dream while unconscious.
- A significant number of subjects woke immediately prior to death. By 'woke' I mean their readings increased from 50 or thereabouts to anything between 70 and 100 and some opened their eyes briefly.

So what does all this mean? It strongly suggests that unconsciousness is not a 'lifeless' or 'mindless' state. It is certainly not the polar opposite of waking consciousness. If anything, it is more akin to sleep for, as happens with sleep, awareness fluctuates and the unconscious subject assimilates and processes information in ways we do not fully understand. They dream, feel pain, hear sounds and appreciate voices. What I do not know is whether anything else happens, and what all this means in the context of death.

The fact that dreaming takes place with people who are unconscious is of more than academic interest. Michael Kearney, a well known and highly respected palliative care doctor, has extensively researched the subject of dreams and healing. He believes that dreams help the sick or dying person prepare for death. This being the case, unconsciousness may in fact be a continuation and ultimately a culmination of this very important preparatory stage.

Although we know very little about dreaming, evidence now suggests it is a state of consciousness in its own right and not some interesting interlude between sleeping and waking. It is a dynamic state full of activity and potential. Dr Michel Jouvet, one of the foremost researchers on the subject of dreams, had a startling revelation, which he describes in his latest book, *The Paradox of Sleep – The Story of Dreaming*. His research has shown that the brain is more active and consumes more energy during the phases of REM (rapid eye movement) sleep – when most dreams occurs – than with ordinary waking consciousness. As evidence now suggests that unconscious dying patients also dream, we can assume their brain is just as active during their dreaming phases. Given that other parts of the body are shutting down, this is somewhat of a paradox and raises questions about what is happening in the mind and brain of those who are dying.

The temporary and dramatic increase in awareness at the moment of death is startling but, given what I have just said, it may not be so unusual after all. The experience of those who care for the dying suggests that this awakening prior to death is not an infrequent occurrence. I have witnessed it on many occasions. These people often stare into space as if looking at something or someone. Whether this is a deathbed vision, part of a dream or a startle response is something we shall discuss shortly.

The findings have major implications for the care we give to those who are dying. It suggests we should relate to them, when unconscious, as though they can hear and, when appropriate, we should include them in our conversations. I always suggest that people introduce themselves when they enter the room of someone who is unconscious, make some form of physical contact (kiss, touch) and tell the person what they are about to do (e.g. brush their hair). A minimum of words is required, as the dying person may not be capable of assimilating everything, just as you can't when you are in a 'dreamy' state. As with sleep, time does not seem to exist for those who are unconscious so don't be concerned about long gaps in conversation or the hours you are away from the bedside. What seems an eternity for you is but a fleeting moment for them.

One reassuring point that came out of the study is that morphine and other medications used appropriately do not significantly alter awareness levels or affect any of the normal processes such as dreaming. Of the twelve people studied, two were on no medication at the time. Their results were remarkably similar to those of the remaining ten, who were on various preparations, including morphine.

Near death experiences and deathbed visions

Altered states of consciousness are not infrequent in the context of dying and most commonly occur within weeks or hours of death. During any of these states individuals are fully aware of their own environment, but have an appreciation of things that others cannot see, hear or experience. Sceptics would call this a hallucination. I believe this is too simple and convenient a label and hope to convince you otherwise.

> *Stella had been near to death for several days. I happened to be in the room when she suddenly sat bolt upright and, with eyes fixed on the wall ahead, beamed with delight. I asked her to describe what she was looking at, but there was no reply. She continued to look ahead as though mesmerised. Her daughter arrived about this time but she, like me, could not distract her mother from what she was experiencing. After several minutes Stella lay back on the bed and died.*

These unusual, but well publicised experiences occur in the face of death or, in the case of NDEs, with the threat of death (note that NDEs and DBVs are very similar and may indeed be the same experience but in different settings). Visions, usually of predeceased relatives and/or religious figures, are the most common and pronounced feature of a DBV and this is nearly always accompanied by a sense of joy and peace that is so overwhelming the person cannot describe it. Given the gravity of the situation these emotions seem out of place. Another striking feature of the visions is their vividness, so much so that the person may awake from sleep or unconsciousness and be totally absorbed and overwhelmed by what they see. According to Drs Karlis Osis and Erlendur Haaraldsson, authors of one large study, the vision is 'so real that only very very rarely will the person doubt the reality of the apparition'.

DBVs and NDEs are not new but the number of reported NDEs has increased dramatically over the last 40 or 50 years. This surge is probably a result of improvements in resuscitation techniques, which have seen many more people survive a life-threatening situation to tell of their experience. Approx-imately 15–50 per cent of people who come close to death recall having an NDE and 25 per cent of those that die will tell of a DBV beforehand. This latter figure may be artificially low, bearing in mind that those who die have fewer opportunities to share their experience.

One of the earliest recorded reports of a DBV concerned a young mother who was dying within days of the birth of her first child. Expecting her patient to be distraught, the doctor was stunned by this woman's apparent peace and sought an explanation. The woman's response to her doctor's leading question was 'If you could see what I can see you would understand'.

In an attempt to find out more about DBVs, we contacted the next of kin of patients who had died in our hospice over a three-month period. We were surprised to learn that 23 per cent had either witnessed their loved one experiencing a DBV or had been told about it by their now deceased relative. In all cases, these visions were described by the dying person, or by the next of kin, as comforting. Comments such as these were common:

- 'Mum said she had seen many of her deceased relatives.'
- 'Mum saw different relatives in the room.'
- 'He saw a person in a white dress holding out her hand.'
- 'She gazed into the air in front of her, whereupon she seemed happy and content.'

Trent was a young man with recently diagnosed but rapidly advancing cancer. The cancer had spread throughout his bones and caused him considerable pain. Despite frequent courses of radiotherapy and large doses of morphine the pain increased, so much so that admission to hospital became necessary. Adjustments to treatment resulted in some, though not complete, pain relief. Despite large doses of morphine he was lucid at all times. He was a popular and well known personality and his room was always filled with visitors. One evening, his father joined the hordes of people in the room and, as he went to sit on the only empty chair, his son called out, 'Be careful you don't sit on my friend, Dad.' 'What friend?' asked his father, looking at the empty chair. 'My friend, a good friend, who will shortly take me away.' Everyone was stunned. Trent then told those present in the room about this friend who had been there with him for several days.

I never got the opportunity to ask Trent about his invisible friend but, in conversation with his family, it seemed as if this 'friend' was not someone he knew or recognised. He was nonetheless a source of comfort during Trent's last days. It would be easy to attribute this to a hallucination, induced by a perilous state of health or a large dose of morphine. Given his otherwise clear mind and appropriate conversation, this proposition seems unlikely. What is important and what really matters is that, in Trent's eyes, this friend was real and brought a quiet and comforting presence during those last few days. Comfort is a theme that characterises many a DBV, as the following example illustrates.

Nina was an elderly Italian woman. She had advanced cancer of the uterus and had been admitted to the local hospice from home. She spoke very little English and, because of this and her weakened state, she made no demands on the staff. She appeared withdrawn and sad. The family had asked she not be told she was dying even though her body language suggested she already knew. One day, just after the family arrived for their regular daily visit, they rushed out of her room, grabbed me as I passed by and urged me to give their mother an injection to settle her. They said she was agitated and was asking to leave the hospice. She was sitting bolt upright in bed, speaking in her native tongue. Her eyes were fixed on the wall as if she was looking at something but what struck me was the broad smile on her face. I asked the family to interpret what Nina was saying. 'I am going on a big holiday, the boat is here, my bags are packed and none of you can come with me.' Although Nina was filled with joy, the family was distraught, as they had interpreted her rambling to mean she wanted to leave the hospice. I explained that she was not asking to leave but was telling her family that the time for her to die had arrived. I encouraged them to sit and let her talk about this journey. She died two days later. Following the funeral, the family returned to the hospice to thank us for caring for their mother and for helping them to understand the significance of Nina's vision.

The next case is more bizarre than most, but the message of comfort that eventually comes as Rhonda hears the words 'It's okay' is equally clear. I was very uncertain about what was happening at the time but trusted my intuition and followed the lead set by Rhonda. Like the other examples, it illustrates the sense of mystery that often prevails around the time of death and how significant events can be easily overlooked, reduced to a mere aberration or placated with medication.

Rhonda had been in the hospice for more than a month with cancer of the bowel. The symptoms of pain and vomiting had been difficult to control and persisted despite numerous changes in medication. I saw her late one morning and asked how things were going. She said she was more comfortable and had not vomited for at least 24 hours. She thanked me for my visit and said she planned to have a sleep.

One hour later I was contacted by the nurse to say that Rhonda was very distressed, rigid with pain and requesting an injection to ease the discomfort. Because this was such a contrast to what I had seen earlier I went to see Rhonda before making a decision on treatment. I found her writhing in pain and clutching a heat pack to her stomach. I knelt by her side and asked her to tell me what was happening. To my surprise, she started speaking in a strange way; her words ran into each other and it was difficult to understand everything she said, but the exchange went something like this.

Rhonda: Oh, it is terrible, all the oranges and browns, like waves, oh, oh.

[She was rigid at this time, appeared frightened and clutched the hot pack tightly to her stomach.]

Michael: Is there any place you can go to get away from them?

Rhonda: Yes, yes, the dark blue. It's beautiful.

Michael: Go to it, Rhonda, and wrap yourself in that dark blue.

[Rhonda relaxed but after a short time spoke again: It's back again, all the oranges and browns. She mentioned other colours that I could not quite catch and again she became very agitated.]

Michael: Go back to the dark blue, Rhonda. It is right by you; wrap yourself tightly in the dark blue.

[Again she relaxed.]

Rhonda: Must get that piping; what's it doing here?

Michael: Tell me about the piping.

Rhonda: What is it doing here?

Michael: Is anyone there with you?

Rhonda: Yes, my aunt [whom she named]. She looks thin and old.

Michael: I think she has come to see how you are. Is anyone else there?

Rhonda: Yes, can't be sure but I think it is her mother.

Michael: Ask them what they want.

[Long silence]

Michael: What did they say, Rhonda?

Rhonda: It's okay.

Michael: Yes, it is okay. All you need to do is stay with the blue and they will look after you.

Rhonda: Jam, I need some blackcurrant jam and blackberry jam.

Michael: I don't have any but will water do?

Rhonda: Yes thanks.

[She had a sip, settled and relaxed into sleep.]

During this exchange Rhonda's eyes were mostly closed. I left the room after she had gone to sleep and a volunteer sat with her. She was still asleep when I returned, one and then two hours later. By the third hour the family had arrived and Rhonda had gone to the bathroom for a wash. At the end of the day the nurses reported that Rhonda was pain-free and comfortable. She was lucid and had a good few hours with her family. As I was about to leave, they asked what magic words I had used! Rhonda died 12 days later having had no further strange episodes. Her death was peaceful, considering the problems associated with her cancer.

These are just a few examples among many that indicate some of the bizarre happenings around death and the comfort dying people can derive from them. It also confirms how little we know or understand about dying and what takes place when someone is dying. Much of the current debate surrounds the possible cause of NDEs, DBVs and other altered states of consciousness. While this is important we must not lose sight of the fact that, whatever the cause, the experience and what it means for that person is what really matters. Looking for causes without appreciating the significance of the experience is similar to studying the roots of a flowering plant while ignoring the flower's beauty.

For the person who is dying, the experience has a deep and powerful meaning that can easily be invalidated or misinterpreted because it is so bizarre to the outsider. Similarly, experiences may be overlooked because they are so subtle. Some of what we label confusion in the dying may in fact be profound experiences that can so easily be lost because we do not tune into the right 'wavelength'. Ram Dass, a well known and respected American psychologist who does a lot of voluntary work for hospices, tells a wonderful story that illustrates this point.

One evening I was contacted by a hospice to see if I could help settle a man who was dying. Despite all manner of medical treatment this man had been 'raving' for days. I sat by the man, who continued to make unintelligible noises. I did not know what was happening or what I should do, but after a while I decided to imitate the sounds. The noise emanating from the room became much louder and the staff wondered if they had done the right thing in calling for outside help. I persisted in imitating the noises and after some time the man turned to me and said, 'So you can see them too?' More of the harmonising followed and the man eventually settled and remained so until his death.

No one really understands what happens during these altered states of consciousness, just as we do not know their cause(s). I have tried to demonstrate that the capacity for awareness in these states is much greater than most of us would believe possible. It is something of a paradox to know that a person's consciousness can expand to incorporate these experiences as they are dying. Some experts suggest that these altered states of consciousness should be called states of superconsciousness; 'super' because of the ability to tune into things that are beyond normal waking consciousness. For the same reason, others have referred to this state as omniconsciousness.

Many who have had an NDE talk of being able to view their body from afar as if it did not belong to them. They have a real sense of living outside the body and, for many, this state was so appealing they had to make a 'conscious' decision to return. Those who have had an NDE say the experience is indescribable and that it feels more real than life itself. So profound is this effect that most lose all fear of death and see life in a totally different light.

Recently, a man dying of a brain tumour told me of the following out-of-body experience (OBE).

> *One afternoon, while sitting in his bed, Chris left his body and sat in a nearby chair. From that position he could see himself lying in the bed, but the person in the chair seemed more real. This person reassured the one in the bed that his children would be okay and well provided for (this, and not the fact he was dying was Chris's major concern). Chris said the conversation lasted one hour and at that point the person in the chair re-entered the body in the bed. He described the experience as peaceful and amazing. While out of his body, Chris had none of the pain or the speech problem that had beset him over the previous month and he was disease-free. Following this out-of-body experience Chris was more at peace, had less pain and was more accepting of his impending death. He died one week later.*

No one can say whether these experiences are machinations of a dying brain or some transcendental event, but whatever the cause there is no doubt they occur. The experiences are hard for us to comprehend and for this reason there is the danger we might reject them as unimportant. Our understanding of unconsciousness and altered states of consciousness – and consciousness for that matter – is rudimentary and any preconceived ideas or biased opinion is not only counterproductive but may also compromise the way we care for those who are dying. What we have learnt about unconsciousness is that we know very little about the experience of dying.

These expanded states of consciousness are not new, nor are they confined to the dying. They have been described by many mystical traditions and for centuries have been an important area of spiritual practice. They may also be induced by ritualistic practices that frequently involve the use of mind-altering substances such as mushrooms. These historical roots have led to a natural conclusion that altered states of consciousness can only be induced, and are not part of a natural state. Recent observations have suggested quite the opposite. Stilling the mind with meditation, prayer, prolonged silence or isolation is now known to be just as potent as ritualistic and spiritual practices in inducing altered states of consciousness.

This raises the possibility that a conscious mind that is both active and interactive, limits consciousness to a state of cognition, and only when it is 'switched off' does it allow the 'wider field' of consciousness to permeate. This is very relevant to dying, particularly when dying includes a period of unconsciousness. Dying introduces physical and mental stillness, social and sensory isolation, conditions known to be conducive to the development of altered states of consciousness. So, not surprisingly, altered states of consciousness, including OBEs, NDEs and DBVs are relatively common among those who are dying. Whether these states are mystical or physiological remains to be determined but their occurrence and significance is now beyond question. If nothing else, the way we care for the dying person who is unconscious bears re-examining.

Irrespective of your belief system, I hope you are now more open to the metaphysical possibilities surrounding death, and appreciate that more rather than less is happening as death approaches. I hope it also gives you the strength and courage to remain close to the one who is dying, to tune into whatever is happening and to speak to them as though they can hear. A prolonged period of unconsciousness may not be as meaningless as many of us previously thought. It may be a necessary incubation and preparation for death.

The best is perhaps what we understand least.

NW CLERK
A Grief Observed

Chapter 7

What happens around the time of death?

The dark and silent river
Pursues through tangled woods a way…

HW LONGFELLOW
The Silent River

Chapter 7

What happens around the time of death?

In an era when few children die and most adults survive beyond the age of seventy years, our idea of death is often constructed from what we see and hear from others and what we are presented through the media. Unless we have been with or cared for someone as they were dying, our concept of death is far removed from the truth and rarely prepares us for the real thing when it comes along. In his autobiography, *In the Face of Death*, Peter Noll speaks of his own experience of dying and says, 'What we figure out in our heads looks quite different once realised in reality'. Only when we face our own death or lose someone we love, will we know death and experience its secrets and its mystery.

The task of being a carer is demanding and unremitting and the roles you need to assume are many and varied. Over the course of a life-threatening illness the tasks and roles change but the goal of maintaining the best quality of life for the one you care for remains the same. As the illness progresses and death approaches, comfort becomes increasingly important, but the uncertainty that has always been there now assumes mammoth proportions as you face countless unknowns. You are no stranger to the unknown but this is different and, no matter how well you have prepared yourself, the occasion will be, as TS Eliot said, 'unexpected when it arrives'.

The time immediately before death and the moment of death are usually the most feared times in the whole process of caring. The many uncertainties, the degree of responsibility and the anguish associated with the occasion make this time arduous and surreal. The responsibility of caring for your loved one as they die can be overwhelming. Their life as well as their death is literally in your hands and, although you will receive enormous support from family, friends, nurses and doctors, you are the one who will be there most of the time and the one likely to be called upon to make decisions. This is never easy and the task is that much harder if this is the first time you have been with someone who is dying and the one you are caring for is very dear to you.

This chapter is written to help you with some of the uncertainties that may arise at 'ground zero' and to throw light on the raft of changes that accompany death or herald its arrival. It deals with the physical changes immediately prior to death and the things that need to be done subsequent to it. I hope it helps you to respond appropriately to these uncertain times, removes some of the anxiety, prepares you for what may happen and empowers you to make decisions in keeping with the wishes of your loved one.

Death is never the same and what is true for one person may not apply to another. The only thing we can say about death is that it is unpredictable in the manner and timing of its arrival. Generalisations can therefore be misleading, so if any of what I say seems irrelevant to your situation, do not think your loved one's dying is out of the ordinary. It may be unique but never out of the ordinary. Every person dies their own death. Often this has parallels with they way they have lived, and just as life can be unpredictable, so too can death. The following comments are therefore to be taken as a guide rather than to be seen as inevitable.

let it go. let it out.
let it all unravel.
let it free and it can be
a path on which to travel

MICHAEL LEUNIG

Predicting the time of death

Death is many things, but never predictable. It may arrive suddenly when you least expect it or, alternatively, dying may be so slow that you wonder if it will ever come. At times, death may seem imminent, and then for no apparent reason the person rallies, leaving you to wonder whether they are in fact dying or whether there is yet some unfinished business. This scenario may be repeated not once but several times. This unpredictable and uncertain course is emotionally draining and makes planning and organising problematic. Most family members want to be present when death occurs and so it is not unusual for them to spend extraordinary amounts of time around the bedside. If this goes on for any length of time, and death seems no closer after several days of waiting, it is reasonable for them, and you the carer, to approach someone (doctor or nurse), ask what is happening and whether earlier plans need to be adjusted.

The best way to handle this situation is to arrange regular meetings with the people involved in your loved one's care. Getting progress reports when death is near allows you to plan ahead. The person you speak to could be the doctor or the nurse and more often than not it will be someone different most days. This can create a problem as everyone, including health care professionals, interprets things differently and some of the messages you are given may be contradictory. If this happens, it is better to point out the discrepancy as there may be a simple explanation.

Asking a doctor or nurse to predict the time of death will not be helpful as the prediction is only a calculated guess based on their experience and what is happening to your loved one at that moment. Getting a prognosis or 'guesstimate' of how long a person may live is, according to Mal and Dianne McKissock, two of Australia's leading authorities on the subject of grief, potentially more harmful than helpful. From my experience, a prognosis creates expectations that may distract people from what is happening each moment. It also creates anxiety that increases as the predicted time approaches. You can only take one hour or one day at a time – things can change so quickly that they render anything that was said one day or several days ago, irrelevant.

This question of prognosis also arises if you or some other person has taken on the responsibility of informing others when death is approaching. Trying to flag the time of death is not only impossible but puts the onus of responsibility on your shoulders, a responsibility you can do without at this time. By all means, pass on information, but the decision when to leave work or to travel can only be made by the individuals themselves. It may be helpful to know that airlines will make every effort to get relatives on the first available flight and will sometimes offer fares at a reduced rate if they are told of the circumstances.

What changes indicate death is near?

The changes I am about to mention are useful markers along the dying trajectory, but remember, their absence does not mean death is still some way removed. Of the many changes that are possible, the following are the best, but not infallible, indicators that death is near:

- unconsciousness
- changes in the pattern of breathing
- changes in the circulation.

Unconsciousness

Death may be sudden and unexpected, but for most it is relatively slow and follows a period of unconsciousness that last hours or days. The nature of unconsciousness is discussed in Chapter 6 but it is worth repeating that unconsciousness is not a state of oblivion but a form of sleep. It does not mean your loved one is unable to hear or respond. Quite the contrary, they may be drowsier than usual and this will ultimately progress to a deep sleep from which they do not awaken. Throughout most of this time, your loved one will be able to hear and their level of awareness is much greater than you could ever imagine.

> *Ian was a strapping 26-year-old man who had battled leukaemia for many years before his ultimate relapse. Knowing he would shortly die he asked that I keep him comfortable and refrain from any heroic measures when the time came. It was only a matter of weeks before he was admitted to the local hospital. He was unconscious from an overwhelming blood infection (septicaemia) and I duly informed the family that he had only hours to live. In keeping with our agreement, I had not commenced any lifesaving measures and arranged that he be kept comfortable.*

The family was distraught, not only because he was dying but also because Ian's much loved sister would not arrive from overseas for four days. Hours and days passed and I was at a loss to explain how someone so ill could live this long. He had not stirred for four days and it was now the day his sister was due to arrive. The very moment she entered the room he opened his eyes and their eyes met. Ian smiled and sighed. He then lapsed back into an unconscious state and died later the same day.

So, yes, unconsciousness is a sign that death is near but whether it is hours or days away cannot be predicted; as we saw with Ian, there are many other factors that put the timing of death beyond our reach. Our study of patients' awareness during states of unconsciousness, described previously, does, however, provide a guide. We noted that the average length of survival from the moment someone became unconscious was three days, with the shortest being one day and the longest eight. Bearing in mind what has already been said about unconsciousness (Chapter 6), use this time to talk to your dying relative, make physical contact and tell them of your movements because they take in much more than you can imagine possible. But try not to count the hours or days.

Breathing

It is not unusual for the pattern of breathing to change in the final hours or days of someone's life. The change may occur in isolation but is more relevant if other changes accompany it. The changes in breathing I am about to describe may not be so significant and should be interpreted carefully in someone with pre-existing lung problems such as emphysema or in those with cardiac disease.

Rapid or irregular breathing is perhaps the most commonly observed change. Breaths may be shallow or vary markedly in depth as well as frequency. There may be periods when breathing stops altogether for as long as 5 to 10 seconds (it will seem longer). The cycle of deep sighing respirations followed by progressively shallow breaths and then no breathing for a few seconds (Cheyne-Stokes respiration) is very common in the late stage of life and a relatively reliable sign that death is near. Please note that this type of breathing can also occur in the sick and elderly who are not dying and its relevance depends on the context in which it appears. With both rapid and irregular breathing there is unlikely to be any associated distress and, although oxygen is often used, it is not essential. So do not feel your loved one's care is compromised if you do not have oxygen in the home.

Sighing respirations – when each breath is accompanied by a distinct sigh, is unnerving and could indicate pain but may also result from the person's position in bed. It is a good idea to notify the nurse or doctor if this pattern of breathing appears, and they will make the necessary assessment and adjustments to your relative/friend's position and treatment. Sometimes the sighing continues despite all measures to ensure your loved one is pain free and well positioned. If this is the case, you can be reasonably confident it is not due to pain or distress, but results from the effort of breathing. Once again, oxygen is not usually required.

Perhaps the most ominous of all breathing patterns is the so-called 'rattly' respiration, where each breath is accompanied by an audible noise, once described to me by a relative as sounding as if the person is breathing underwater. The noise results from air passing through secretions that have accumulated in the back of the throat and/or the breathing tubes. As disturbing as it may sound, your relative/friend is by this stage deeply unconscious and almost certainly beyond feeling pain or distress. The fact that they do not cough when so much fluid is present in their throat serves to confirm the absence of distress. This form of breathing occurs only in those who are very close to death, so close that the breathing is labelled 'death rattles'.

Very little can be done to reduce the noise and, while doctors and nurses know it is not distressing for the person dying, they realise this is anything but true for those present. For that reason, an essential part of the treatment is to remind and reassure family that their loved one has no awareness of what is happening. Repositioning sometimes helps and a drug called hyoscine may be administered in an attempt to dry the secretions. Hyoscine helps sometimes, but not always. Suction is equally ineffective as most of the secretions are too far down the breathing tubes to be reached. Oxygen is frequently given but is not essential.

Rattly respiration usually means that death is only minutes or hours away and family that wish to be present at the time of death should be notified. It is not necessary to call a doctor or nurse but most families do, if only to be reassured that all that needs to be done is being done. Noisy breathing may occur outside of the deathbed situation in people with chronic lung or heart conditions. The main difference being, these people are conscious at the time. The need for assessment and treatment then depends on whether this is a sudden or relatively recent change and the level of distress the person experiences at the time. Ring your doctor or nurse if you are unsure.

Circulation

As someone edges closer to death the lips, fingers and toes often become bluish and the backs of the hands, forearms and shins develop a mottled appearance. They may be more sweaty than usual and the pulse, by this time, is very weak and often impossible to feel. All these signs indicate the circulation is now very sluggish and death is near. If these changes occur in association with rattly breathing, death may be only minutes away.

Bearing in mind the emphasis placed on pulse and blood pressure in the hospital situation, family may wonder why these 'vital signs' are not checked when someone is dying. The reason is simple: pulse and blood pressure tell us no more and often less about a situation than observation alone. Not only are blood pressure and pulse rate readings unnecessary, they are often difficult to measure when someone is dying. More importantly, they reduce death to a biological event rather than a human experience. One way we can respect the significance of the occasion is be fully present and not distracted by unimportant things such as the 'vital signs'. Dying is not a medical condition that needs to be monitored, it is a defining time in people's lives, and so the less interference the better.

How can someone so sick survive so long?

Dying can be slow, with no measurable change from one day to the next. There may be times when you wonder if your loved one is really dying, whether medication is prolonging the dying or if there is some unfinished business that is keeping them alive. You may find it hard to conceive how anyone so sick can continue to live, particularly if they are not eating and drinking. You may also be physically and emotionally exhausted and, as much as you love and will miss the one who is dying, you may think it is time for them to go and for their suffering to end. Ultimately, you become caught in an impasse – part of you hopes death will come soon, but another part dreads the very thought.

This way of thinking is not harsh nor does it reflect unfavourably on you. It is not heartless to want your loved one's suffering to end. My impression is that most carers, relatives and friends engage in this silent discourse but, believing it to be dispassionate, they keep it to themselves and suffer in silence. Talking about the impasse puts you in touch with your feelings, releases some of the emotional charge and dissipates some of the grief.

The ultimate act of dying is thought to involve some form of letting go – letting go of the people and all the things that are loved and, ultimately, letting go of life. The act of letting go can be much harder for some than for others. There is also a need for family and friends to let go. The dying person can sometimes sense your 'hanging on' and death can be protracted for this very reason.

From the dying person's perspective there may be fears or unfinished business that causes them to hang on to life. They may also need affirmation from those they love and reassurance that it is okay to die. Unfinished business may involve saying goodbye to someone (as with Ian), or surviving to partake of a special event, as was the case with Pam (see Chapter 6). So, if someone's death seems to be taking longer than expected, consider all these possibilities and do whatever needs be done to address them.

Giving people permission to die is a beautiful gift. To hear family say how much the person is loved, how much they have meant to their life, how much they will be missed but never forgotten is not unlike the loving embrace we give to a child as we put them to bed. It relaxes the dying person and helps them to complete this necessary journey. Say these things as often as you feel necessary and invite all members of the family to do likewise.

Occasionally, death may come suddenly and unexpectedly. Stories of family leaving a sickroom to make a cup of tea only to return and discover their relative has died are not uncommon. In most cases, this can be put down to the unpredictable nature of the illness but sometimes there is some connection between the two events. My belief is, there is a right time to die and, whether that death is earlier or later than anticipated, there is always a reason for it. Often we are not privy to the reason, but it helps our grief and erases some of the 'whys' if we can make space for this possibility. So, accepting that we do not know the hour or the day, make sure you and others say their goodbyes and share with their loved one, whether unconscious or not, everything that needs to be said. That way, if death comes unexpectedly you will not be left with that dreaded thought 'If only I had said...'

What can you do as death approaches?

This is a tough time for you and your family. Apart from ensuring your dying relative/friend is comfortable and pain free, be gentle with yourself, recognise your needs and the needs of those close to you, particularly children. Get as much rest as your body demands. You may not want to leave the room or the house but time to sleep, catch your breath, walk in nature or sit quietly on your own can be restorative and help you overcome the bumps along the way. If you and your family decide to do a 24-hour vigil, I strongly recommend this be on a roster basis to ensure the load is divided equally and that each has enough rest and/or time away to recuperate.

By now all medication given by mouth will have ceased and only that essential for comfort will be administered (by injection under the skin or by means of a syringe driver). This usually includes morphine or some other analgesic, an anti-emetic if nausea has been a problem and a sedative. Morphine is continued because pain does not disappear when someone is close to death and is often given in combination with a sedative to ensure comfort. Oxygen is required only if breathing has been or is a problem.

The syringe driver is a battery-driven device that delivers the day's medication from a syringe into the tissue beneath the skin via a 'butterfly' needle (a thin plastic tube). This is a safe, painless and effective way of administering essential medications that can no longer be taken by mouth.

As bodily pain may arise from being in one position for long periods it is recommended that you turn your relative from one side to another every four to six hours during the day and less frequently at night. Always ensure their arms and legs are well positioned and cushions are placed between bony prominences. Rubbing the back and limbs after repositioning soothes discomfort, and is another means of making intimate contact. Of course, as death nears, the need for turning diminishes.

Your loved one will have stopped eating well before this time, but the mouth still needs to be kept moist almost to the very end. If incontinence pads are in place these should be changed when wet or soiled. Again, you may be surprised at the amount of urine someone can pass when they are dying. If a urinary catheter is in place, the volume of urine will diminish over time and the urine will become concentrated (darker in colour). Bowels are most unlikely to open, but if restlessness occurs, constipation (and a full bladder) is one of many possible problems that should be excluded. Regular bed baths are necessary to maintain cleanliness, comfort and dignity. They are usually done by the visiting nurse(s), but if you prefer to do it, they would be very happy to show you how. Alternatively, you can do it together. Don't however, feel obliged to take on any more than you can physically or emotionally cope with.

Continue to clean and dress all skin wounds daily or as often as is required and change the bed linen and pyjamas to maintain dignity and hygiene. Within reason, do what you can to keep the room free of flies and insects as these can be more than a mere irritation to someone who is unconscious or too weak to fan them away.

Ensure you have the phone numbers of all key people and keep the list in a conspicuous place. Always check your doctor's availability after hours and at weekends, and if they have made themselves available, add their home or mobile phone number to your list. When death is near, it is advisable to speak to the doctor before each weekend to fill them in on the situation and to ensure they will be around. If the doctor is unavailable, but is linked to an after-hours or emergency medical service, get that number(s) and ask the doctor to inform the service of the situation. If the doctor is unavailable and is not linked to an after-hours service, you will need to get the name and number of a doctor or service who will visit in times of emergency or death.

How will I know when death occurs?

This may seem an unusual question but it is very relevant if you have no formal first aid training and are caring for your loved one at home alone. From a medical and legal perspective a person is dead when breathing stops and no heartbeat is audible with a stethoscope. You will know your relative has died by the absence of breathing. It sounds simple but may not be for any number of reasons:

- Breathing may be so shallow immediately before death it is hard to know when it stops.
- Some people continue to take tiny gasps even though effective breathing has ceased. This gasping may go on for many minutes.
- You may be too upset or feel unable to make the assessment.
- If your vision is poor and you are alone it may be hard to determine if breathing has stopped.

Whatever the situation, just remember you do not have to make a decision or act immediately. If you think your loved one has died, but are not certain, just sit there until it becomes clear that breathing has stopped. Alternatively, if you are too upset or feel unable to do this, call for help. If you are alone, ring a friend or relative. You could also ring the doctor or nurse if you prefer.

What should I do immediately after my loved one has died?

This is a very special moment. Sit by your loved one and spend whatever time you need to take in the situation and to say goodbye. You may offer a prayer, light a candle, place some flowers on or beside the body or perform a ritual in keeping with your cultural or spiritual beliefs. Short readings from a book or text such as the Bible or the Koran recognise the significance of the occasion and may offer solace to those present at the time. I have found selected readings from The Prophet (see Bibliography) both appropriate and meaningful.

It is okay to touch, kiss and cuddle the person just as it is to speak to them. When you are ready, ring the doctor or nurse. If death occurs in the early hours of the morning, you can defer phoning for several hours, either for your sake or their convenience. Do what you are most comfortable with.

Do not ring for an ambulance and do not ring 000. Either of these calls could result in the ambulance officers instituting cardio-pulmonary resuscitation (CPR) unless there is documentation to the contrary. Any form of resuscitation at this time is futile and a most undignified way for your loved one to end their life.

At some convenient time, carry out the following tasks:

- Turn off the oxygen and remove the mask or prongs.
- Lay the body flat with one pillow under the head.
- Remove all blankets.
- Turn off any electric blanket and room heating.
- Phone the doctor and nurse.

What happens after a person dies?

After you have phoned the doctor and nurse, several things follow. The doctor will confirm that your loved one has died, and will complete the necessary death and cremation (if required) certificates. These procedures are necessary before the body can be removed. The certificate(s) are given to the funeral director when they come to collect your loved one's body. Official copies of the death certificate are only available through the Registry of Births, Deaths and Marriages in your state or territory (see Appendix) and will be required to claim on life insurance or superannuation policies or to settle other financial or property transactions. For further information on death certificates, see Chapter 13, 'Practical matters to ponder'.

The nurses will remove all items of medical equipment attached to your relative, such as the syringe driver, butterfly needles or catheters, and will then wash the body. You may, if you wish, do this yourself or help the nurses. This is a form of ritual that may ultimately help your grieving.

After the wash, your relative will be dressed in fresh nightwear or attire that you and/or your loved one may have chosen before the death. I always encourage families to choose clothes that in some way identify the person and to do the dressing themselves. Many a time I have sat in a nearby room as this was being done and, in almost all cases, heard crying and laughter as family reminisce about the person and events that led them to choose that attire. The ritual is cathartic and every family that did it was pleased they had done so. The type of clothing and accessories never ceased to amaze me. It has included scuba diving gear, golf attire (including shoes and putter), torn jeans, Hawaiian shirts, hiking boots, jogging shoes, favourite pyjamas, bright lipstick and expensive perfumes.

The funeral director should be notified about the death and a time negotiated for them to come to remove the body. The laws pertaining to how long you may keep your loved one at home after death and before burial or cremation have been relaxed, and are things you can negotiate with the funeral director at the time of the initial contact. For this and other reasons I recommend you make contact with the funeral director of your choice early rather than late in the course of the illness. This also allows your dying relative to have a say, if they so choose.

The time between death and when the funeral director comes is precious and may be used in whatever way you choose. Depending on your beliefs and customs, it may be a time for prayer and ritual or a time to reflect on the life of the deceased person. Saying goodbye can be awkward and difficult. Numbness, exhaustion and disbelief can overtake you at this time and if you are in the room with others you may be a little reticent about saying publicly what you feel. I recommend that each family member and close friend spend a little time alone with the person who has died to say goodbye and share with them anything they may wish or need to say. This can be emotional but it is a moment you will treasure for years to come.

Are you certain they are dead?

There are many reasons why people ask this question. The commonest is disbelief. Even though death has been expected for some time it seems so unreal when it ultimately comes. Some family members will only believe it after death as been confirmed by a person with some credibility such as a doctor or nurse. Others need extra reassurance their loved one has died for fear they may be buried alive. If this concerns you, ask for and get the reassurance you need, otherwise the thought may haunt you over the days and weeks that follow. The absence of breathing and a heartbeat for a period of one minute is an absolute sign that death has occurred. Your doctor will make certain of this before completing the necessary certificates.

Confirmation of death also gives you permission to grieve openly and to express emotions that may have been held in check during the last days of the illness. It is thus a release, but also a surreal realisation that the person has died and that your life will be forever different. CS Lewis describes it as like losing a leg – part of you has been taken away.

Should we involve the children?

How should children be told? Should they see the dead person? Should they attend the funeral/cremation? There is no simple answer to these questions. Circumstances surrounding the death, family beliefs, customs, the children's ages, their relationship to the person who has died and their wishes will all influence the ultimate choice. If you get the opportunity and have the emotional strength, try and deal with these questions earlier rather than later. Doing it this way ensures the children are involved, helps them to understand what is happening and gives them opportunities to ask questions and talk about how they feel. This is particularly relevant if it is the child's parent or sibling who is dying. A child's reaction is unpredictable, so do not be alarmed if they are extremely distressed or, at the other extreme, unaffected, for neither of these or any state in between is abnormal.

When a child is to be informed about the death it is preferable that this be done by someone very close to them and in a place where they feel safe enough to cry and express their emotions. Inform the child clearly and directly about what has happened. Don't be afraid to use the word 'dead' or 'death'. Euphemisms should be avoided, as these only create confusion in their mind. Give them adequate time to take in what you have said and to ask questions. Don't be misled by a prolonged silence, or the absence of tears.

Children's responses are totally unpredictable and may range from an apparent lack of interest to aggressive behaviour. Don't misinterpret this, as it may be the only way the child can show their grief. Depending on the response, cuddle them or give them space, but, most importantly, give them time. Then and only then, ask them if they would like to accompany you to say goodbye to the dead person. Again, give them time to ponder their answer. If it happens to be 'no', check with them a little later to make sure they have not changed their mind. If they say 'yes', prepare them gently for what they will see and what they may like to say. Then, hand in hand, lead them slowly into the room, halting if they seem to baulk, reassuring them you will go slowly and that there is no rush. Once there, give them whatever time they need, but watch for the non-verbal cues. Generally, children cope much better with death than we give them credit for.

Whether children should attend the funeral/cremation will depend on many of the factors outlined above. Providing the children are old enough and there are no unusual circumstances, my habit has been to encourage families to let the children decide. When it comes to grief, children often take their cues from the adults and, if you consider it natural and normal for them to attend the funeral, so will they. Children may feel overlooked if they are excluded from this ritual. To be looked after by friends or neighbours when they know other family members are attending the funeral can be very unsettling and leave them with unanswered questions.

Adult family members are naturally concerned about exposing children and adolescents to situations they believe to be too traumatic or unsettling. There is, however, recent evidence from the United States that suggests not all children respond in the way that we adults expect. Many children experience positive outcomes or what the researchers term, 'post-traumatic growth' in response to stressful situations such as a parent being diagnosed with or dying of cancer. One of the major factors in preventing distress and creating resilience was the availability of information about their parent's cancer or the events that ensued including death. These children are thought to grow up with a greater awareness of life and death and make life choices that suggest they appreciate life more than they fear death.

Chapter 8

Care of a child

Gradually, I began to see
that the story was still unfolding;
rather than ending with Hannah's death,
it had only begun.

MARIA HOUSDEN
Hannah's gift

Chapter 8

Care of a child

This chapter looks at the wide-ranging challenges that invariably arise when a child or adolescent is dying. This tragic situation is now, fortunately, much less common in western countries than it once was. In the early part of the twentieth century every family could expect one or more of their children to die but now, in developed countries at least, the number of infants under the age of one year that dies is extremely small. Unfortunately, the same cannot be said for children from indigenous cultures, poorer nations and developing countries, where infant mortality remains unacceptably high and the death of a child before teenage years is relatively common.

Paediatric palliative care specialist Dr John Collins, writing in *Death and Dying in Australia*, said that in 1997 throughout Australia there were 1341 deaths of infants below the age of one year and 726 deaths of children aged between one and 14 years of age. This is a remarkable turnaround from 100 years ago. Similar improvements have been recorded in most developing countries and, while this is a reassuring trend, it is small consolation for parents whose child has died or for those whose child is dying. If anything, it adds to a parent's grief: knowing their child is one of a very small number that die each year.

Given these statistics, there are relatively few doctors, nurses or other professional people with experience in the care of dying children – I have cared for only a handful over the last 40 years. The death of our daughter, however, taught me more than I could ever have gleaned as a doctor, and much of what I have to say comes from that one experience.

In this chapter I also discuss the special needs of children when someone close to them dies – a sibling, parent or grandparent, for example. These scenarios are more frequent than the death of a child. Depending on who it is that dies and the circumstances, that death could be one of the most traumatic events a child is ever likely to face, with emotional and behavioural repercussions that go on for years. On this matter I draw heavily on other people's experience as my involvement with bereft children is often limited to a relatively brief time before and after the death. As you can imagine, many of the issues arise well after this time when, as with adults, the reality of the loss hits home.

The dying child

In all but the very young, children with a life-threatening illness do have some insight into their situation and the concept they form of their illness and their fate is pieced together from many sources. Unremitting symptoms, frequent tests, hospitalisations, the effects of treatment, the sight of others like them and their ever contracting world convince them that something is not right. This, together with the messages they receive, the behaviour of others towards them and the observation that their life has not only changed, but that it is different from that of their siblings and friends, leads them to conclude that all is not as it should be.

How and when this progresses to an appreciation of death and the knowledge that they are indeed dying is impossible to know. Children, like adults, live in the hope that what they go through will make things right. They suffer all this, not only hoping they will improve but often to satisfy doctors and family who reinforce the need for treatment for exactly the same reason. To see your child suffer is extremely traumatic but the alternative, death, is almost more than any parent can endure.

Kids are very astute and when things are not going well they pick up the subtle cues just as well, if not better, than adults. At some deep level they become aware of their fate even though it may not have been conveyed to them in words. Like adults, they frequently know more than they say. Dr Elisabeth Kübler-Ross spent a lot of time working with children who were dying of cancer. Many of these children had not been told about their illness or that they were dying. Almost all, however, were aware that they were dying and, while many lacked the verbal skills and/or the opportunity to say what they felt, they depicted it accurately and vividly in drawings or play. One drawing, done by a young child with an undisclosed (to the child) brain tumour, featured a large 'lump' on the side of his head. Not only did he know about the tumour, the drawing localised the tumour to its exact position, and other parts of the drawing gave a clear message that he knew he was dying.

What death means to any child is little short of guesswork. Many hypotheses exist but they are only guides and do not tell us what it is like for any individual child. This is, of course, equally true for adults. Children don't have a well formulated view about death – in fact, for them it is hazy and incomprehensible. On the other hand, they do have a lot of unanswered questions that they are often afraid to ask or do not know how to ask. Even though they may not understand, most appreciate that death results in some form of separation from those they love and, like adults, their fear is of the unknown – they fear death just as they fear the dark. This analogy not only helps us understand how children perceive death but also how you as a parent can best help them confront the unknown.

The last child I cared for was a young girl aged five years who had been sick for much of her short life. Neva's life revolved around hospitals, tests and treatments and all of that must have been as frightening to her as any dark lonely night. Her parents accompanied her through all of this and their presence no doubt gave her the courage to face the 'dark'. When treatment was no longer effective and the endless round of visits to the doctor, tests and treatment had ceased, attempts were made to prepare her for her inevitable death. While I was not present as that delicate matter was explored, I visited her many times afterwards and during those visits it became clear that death for her meant separation from those she loved, and what she feared most was the thought of being all alone in a coffin. This knowledge was enormously painful for the parents to hear and for any five-year-old to bear, particularly as she had rarely been alone at any time in her life.

How do you talk to a dying child?

There will be no shortage of advice about how to talk to your child about illness and death. Everyone has an opinion and these opinions, even those of the so-called experts, are often conflicting and frequently add to your confusion. By all means, listen to what the experts have to say but trust your own intuition and think twice about doing something that does not feel right. The relationship between a child and a parent is as unique as it is special and your child will seek to recapture as much of this as possible during times of illness. With all the changes that illness brings, one of the few things that remains stable and gives a certain security is your love and the relationship that has been forged over the years.

What your child needs most throughout their illness is your presence and your love. You may at times feel overwhelmed by all that is happening or unsure how to respond to challenging situations or probing questions. This is normal. You cannot make things better and there are no right answers, but remember that nine-tenths of communication is non-verbal and so it is the quality of your relationship and not what you say or do that matters. Given this, the following pieces of information, gathered from a variety of experts, may be helpful.

As a parent, your focus in dealing with your sick child is always to try to make things better. You relieve pain, soothe aches, and provide nourishment for the body and nurturing for the soul. You do whatever you can and often go to extraordinary lengths to ensure your child's needs are met. With the prospect of death there is little else you can do, but follow Dylan Thomas's entreaty and 'Do not go gentle into that good night/ Rage, rage against the dying of the light'.

Death is not a problem that can be solved and in the case of a young child it is an outcome that we all dread and hope never to face. To have your child predecease you is confronting and painful. According to an ancient Chinese legend, the greatest blessing that can be bestowed on any family is to have the oldest die first and for no child to predecease their parent. The challenge you face or have already faced is the move from trying to solve problems to just listening. In his book *Care of the Soul*, Thomas Moore puts this in perspective when he says:

> *The basic intention in any caring, physical or psychological, is to alleviate suffering. But in relation to the symptom itself, observation means first of all listening and looking carefully at what is being revealed in the suffering.*

We are referring to your child's suffering and you being there for them, but the same is also true for you. To have someone who can do for you what you do for your child is a blessing for which you will be eternally grateful.

So how do you comfort a child in the shadow of death? In his book, *Death, Grief and Mourning*, John Stephenson quotes the wonderful work of Myra Bluebond-Langer, who emphasises the loneliness of dying children as they try to protect their parents, while parents at the same time 'defend their child against the awful truth'. Such collusion serves only to isolate one from the other – the child dies with both parties knowing this will happen yet unable to share their deepest feelings, which become more painful the longer they are locked away.

We feel loneliness only when we run from it.

ROLLO MAY
Love and Will

Running from our fears not only intensifies our loneliness but also adds to a child's fear. This running may take on forms other than avoidance. It can be disguised in futile attempts to solve all the problems or by efforts to make things better. Thomas Moore urges us just to be there, to be honest and as vulnerable as the situation demands ('just' does not imply this is easy). Allowing a child to determine the course of a conversation often results in prolonged and painful silences. These are not vacuums where nothing happens, but quite the opposite. They are the times when children search for what is in your heart and mind and, not infrequently, if given the time they will ask a profound question or make some revealing comment. So:

- Allow your child to determine the pace and content of the communication.
- Avoid meetings set up for the sole purpose of talking about death. This often results in more rather than less pain for all concerned. Not that the topic should be avoided, but only that there is a time and a place for it. You as a parent will know when that time is right.
- When the topic of death comes up, allow your child to explore their concept of death at their own pace. Listen carefully to what they say and observe their body language. Answer all relevant questions honestly and as best you can.
- Do not be afraid to show emotion as this may free your child to do likewise; it lets them know, rather than suspect, what their illness means for you. Children and teenagers understand the language of emotions better than words.
- If you talk about or show your pain, remember to reassure your

child that they are not responsible and you do not hold them to blame.

- Tell them how much you love them and how much they mean to you.
- Explore realistic ways of dealing with your child's fears and concerns. The young girl, Neva, that I spoke of earlier in this chapter was not frightened by death per se but by separation and the thought of her (her body) being all alone in an enclosed coffin. This was an equally painful thing for her parents to hear but, among tears and much angst, they explored this and other fears. What started out as a dreaded subject became the catalyst for a moving and healing dialogue between parents and child.
- Give whatever time is necessary for dialogue, but ensure wherever possible that time and space is made for the 'normal' things in a child's life. Like any adult, kids with a life-threatening illness oscillate between a world of sickness (with the fear of death) and one of relative normality. When they are into the normal things of life they do not need to be reminded of death. There will always be plenty of time for that. 'Normality' is as precious for them as it is for adults.
- Uncharacteristic behaviour and/or emotional outbursts all have a root cause. They are a cry for help.
- Make time for and be aware of the needs of other children in the family.
- Make sure the school and the parents of your child's best friends know what is happening. These friends are often pivotal in your child's support network and frequently seek and need support from their own parents, teachers or school counsellors.

The difficulty lies
not in solving problems
but in expressing them.

TEILHARD DE CHARDIN

How should pain be treated?

It goes without saying that a child's physical comfort should be maintained to the best of our ability throughout the course of their illness. Children may not complain, even when pain or other symptoms are present. They may struggle to decribe how they feel and, when they do, it can be hard for someone else to appreciate the level of their discomfort. Physical pain may manifest as a behavioural problem, restlessness, disturbed sleeping or emotional withdrawal. The younger the child the greater is the barrier to effective communication. Adults who are dying frequently underplay their symptoms and carers, including doctors, underestimate their complaints. There is every reason to believe the same is true, possibly more so, with children. Recent evidence, in fact, suggests that almost 50 per cent of hospitalised children have moderate or severe unrelieved pain that is either unrecognised or undertreated. This being the case, we should give children the benefit of any doubt and consider a trial of treatment or increased doses of treatment if we suspect they have pain.

The question of treatment is far from simple. Not only do we have the problem of assessing symptoms, there is the added concern that no parent wants their child to have 'drugs' if they are not absolutely necessary. Such a dilemma can only be resolved by discussing the pros and cons of medication with your doctor. I would generally recommend a trial of treatment if there is any doubt. If the drug happens to be morphine, all the myths and misconceptions about its safety and dangers come to the surface. What was said in Chapter 3 about morphine and the adult patient is equally true for a child. If morphine is being considered this may be a good time to review that information.

Should we persevere with food?

The question of food and fluids is the same for children as it is for adults. Give them what they want and only when they want it. Fluids help to keep the mouth and throat moist, reducing discomfort and the risk of throat infections. Fluids of any type will suffice so be guided by your child's fancies. Ice blocks do the job perfectly well and are often looked upon as a treat. At this stage in your child's illness, appetite may be poor and food may make them feel less well than they are already. Offer food by all means, but do not be surprised if they say no. If they do want food, give them what they want in small amounts – the sight of a large serving may be enough to turn them off eating. Psychologically, it is better that they ask for more rather than struggle with and leave a larger serve partly eaten.

Intravenous or subcutaneous fluids are rarely indicated even when your child stops eating or drinking altogether. Fluids given in this way have negligable nutritional or life-sustaining value and may result in unwanted side effects. Children with a life-threatening illness do not die of starvation or dehydration but from the effects of their disease. They do not feel hungry and, if they do feel thirsty, the only way this can be eased is by keeping the mouth and lips moist.

Do deathbed visions (DBVs) or near death experiences (NDEs) occur with children?

The question of whether children experience deathbed visions and near death experiences has been examined by many people, including the Australian researcher Cherie Sutherland. Her work clearly shows that children do have NDEs and that they are very similar to those experienced by adults. Because of the similarities between NDEs and DBVs it is reasonable to assume the latter also occur. Dr Elisabeth Kübler-Ross certainly thought so and often gave examples of children describing visions in which they saw and named pre-deceased relatives. As a parent it is comforting to know that these types of experiences are thought to occur as frequently with children as they do with adults.

> *Neva often slept with her parents in their generous king-size bed. One morning, as her father got up to make a cup of tea,*

he noticed Neva seemingly wide awake but with her eyes fixed on an open window. He was quite surprised when she did not respond to his morning greeting and her gaze remained unbroken as he walked through her field of vision. She looked so peaceful he decided not to disturb her, and went into the kitchen. When he returned a few minutes later and went to greet Neva, he was shocked to find she had died. Her death was not unexpected but the timing surprised him. Only minutes before she had appeared more awake and peaceful than for some time.

Days later when Neva's father was reflecting on this event, he said it appeared as if she was staring at something. He was not aware of anything unusual other than her fixed gaze and her apparent serenity. She appeared to be looking at something, but what, we will never know. Neva did not talk a lot about her dying but I suspect she knew death was imminent. Late in her illness she asked her family to care for her much loved puppy and to make sure it was registered. I was there at the time and this request had all the hallmarks of attending to unfinished business.

Your grief

Throughout this chapter I have referred to the enormous grief parents feel when one of their children is dying. There must be very few life events that have such a profound and long-lasting effect as the death of a child.

Your grief starts the moment you first suspect or become aware of your child's illness. From that time on it is a roller coaster road with any number of things adding to or appeasing your concerns. These include news about your child's progress, test results, changes in treatment, new or worsening symptoms, the way doctors or nurses relate to you and the way people do or don't acknowledge you. The flavour of your grief is not only influenced by all these outside events but also by who you are and how you deal with crises. The importance of this lies in the realisation that you cannot compare your grief with that of others. If you have a spouse or a partner it is very likely you will be in different 'spaces' for much of the time. This can put a strain on the best of relationships and, if the uniqueness of grief is not appreciated, unrealistic expectations and added tensions will surely arise.

If other children are involved they, too, grieve for the loss of their brother or sister and for the loss of the security and stability that existed beforehand. More than ever they need your love and reassuring presence. They also need to know they are not to blame for what is happening to their sibling or for your grief; nor should they feel bad about wanting things to return to normal.

Can anything be done to help me in my grief?

There will be days when you feel life is not worth living and you cannot bear to face another day. This is not unexpected or unusual and, while it may be hard to believe now, this cloak of blackness will ultimately lift. The pain of your loss will always be there but you and your way of life will return to a semblance of normality at some unpredictable time in the future. Anniversaries and other reminders will always provoke intense sadness, but over time the wounds will heal, although a scar will always remain. Grief does not like to be contained and there is plenty of evidence to suggest that those who express their grief fare much better physically and psychologically than those who do not show or talk about the way they feel. The finer points about living with grief are covered in the Chapters 11 and 12, but a few things are worth repeating now.

As grief starts from the moment your child's diagnosis is made, and sometimes before, whatever you can do from that moment on is helpful. That may involve unburdening yourself with your spouse/partner and/or best friends, and finding space outside the 'sickroom' that you can escape to when the need arises. What you do is a matter for you to decide but the important thing is to do something and not to be inhibited by a sense of obligation or feelings of guilt. This may not be appropriate if death is imminent or during times of crisis, but if the illness is chronic, then time to yourself can help you as well as the quality of the relationship with your child, partner and other children. You need to give yourself permission to do this – if you don't, who will?

Communication is often the means used to resolve or prevent problems but, with grief, there is no solution. In your situation the purpose of communication is not to solve problems but to unburden yourself. It involves telling others how you feel and knowing those people hear what you say. You may feel terrible in the process but the release is a safety valve for emotions that would otherwise build up and possibly explode. It also helps the other person(s) appreciate a little of how you feel.

The position is reversed when your sick child, spouse/partner or other children talk to you. This can be painful and challenging at the best of times but is worse when you are intimately involved with what is happening and have hardly enough emotional reserve for yourself, let alone for those who are unburdening. You can usually sense whether this is a crucial time, a time to stop and attend, but if you are unsure, give them the benefit of the doubt. 'Intuition is the voice of the soul,' says the inspirational author Gary Zukav and, if we listen to it, it rarely lets us down.

Say everything that needs to be said

After your child dies there will always be the inevitable regrets but the ones that hurt the most are thoughts about things you wanted to say but didn't. Opportunities to do this cannot be made, they just happen, and they usually happen at the most unlikely times, like the middle of the night. The things you and your child may wish to say can only be spoken if the environment is right – not just the physical environment but the emotional and spiritual climate, too. Your task is to continually create a micro-environment where this can happen and, if it does, that is wonderful. If it doesn't, then what you have created may have been enough for your child to know what is within your heart. The language of intuition is the native tongue of any child.

Children have great intuitive sense and if they are not too sick they will ask the important questions at the right time. But be prepared, as the question may be blunt or somewhat obtuse. It is a matter of tuning into their wavelength, being absolutely honest with your answers and avoiding as much as possible the use of euphemisms. When it comes to an understanding of death, children are no more and no less wiser than adults, but they do know when we are being evasive. If you don't know the answer, say so, and throw the question back, asking what he/she thinks. What starts off as an innocuous inquiry may develop into a deep and meaningful dialogue. What children often seek is an opportunity to talk rather than an answer to their question.

Honouring your child's life and death

Death may be forbidding and frightening but the time immediately before and after death provides opportunities for you to honour your child. These opportunities will not ease the pain, but they may free you from some of the helplessness that prevails. The thought of honouring someone around the time of their death is not new and in times past this took the form of rituals. Unfortunately, rituals have all but disappeared from western society and those that remain run the risk of becoming mere formalities. This is in stark contrast to 'less' developed and eastern countries which maintain rich traditions and rituals around death.

Here are a few things you might like to consider:

- Do all you possibly can to ensure your child dies 'well'. That may include a pain-free death or dying at home; if the latter is not possible, ensure the hospital/hospice environment is as you and your child would want.
- Do what you can to ensure your child does not die alone. This is something you cannot achieve on your own: you will need to

enlist the support of others. Despite all the best laid plans, your child may still die just at that moment when no one is present. This can be devastating, particularly if you have done everything to assure otherwise. I like to think there is a reason for this happening and I believe that, in some strange way, it is a child's final gift to the family.

- Plan some form of ritual for when your child dies. This may take the form of readings, stories, music or song. Partake in the washing and the laying out that follow death and invite other members of the family to be part of this (if they so choose). Dress your child in their favourite clothes and put a favourite toy/item beside or on their body.
- Light a candle and keep your child at home for as long as you choose. This is possible and is something you can negotiate with the funeral director.
- Plan a burial or cremation that celebrates their life and acknowledge openly how they have enriched your life.

Further down the track you may find a cause you wish to pursue that is in some way related to your child's death. This is by no means the norm but for some it becomes another way of finding meaning in what has happened. After our daughter died of SIDS my wife and I became active members of the SIDS Association, and for some years acted as the local support people for others who had a cot death. A friend whose son was killed in a motor vehicle accident lobbied hard and long to have certain police procedures changed. All these things may seem insignificant, yet they are important; in some small way they put meaning back into life, which death otherwise threatens to remove completely.

Almost everything you do will seem insignificant,
but it is important that you do it.

MAHATMA GANDHI

How can I be there for my other children?

Depending on their age, children have varying levels of understanding as to what is happening with their sick sibling. They may be unaware of the details of the illness or that their sibling is dying but, as a general rule, you should assume they know more than appearances and behaviour would otherwise suggest. If they do know their sibling is dying, their concept of death is unlikely to be as you would imagine. Depending on their age it could be either non-existent, rather simplistic like a sleep, or a frightening figure that takes people away (and can therefore 'get' them too). Alternatively, they may have an adult concept where death means the end of life as they know it.

What children know is that things have changed within the home. There may be many more visitors, parents may spend less time with them and more with their sick sibling (or whoever is sick). They also note but fail to understand why their parents who were once happy and playful are now sad and cry a lot, and they wonder if they are responsible. There may be less time for the usual outings, stories and games. Noise and laughter are now strangely absent. Meal times are different, television is no longer banned and the phone never stops ringing. Everything around them is different, but the reason is what intrigues and concerns them.

Kids do not welcome this type of change and will attempt to maintain or restore what has been normal for them. They will want to play and may use games to draw you back into their life. If this fails they may resort to attention-seeking behaviour. Drs John Collins, a Palliative Care Physician at the Westmead Children's Hospital in Sydney and John Stephenson, Associate Professor of Sociology at San Diago State University in the USA both say: 'Children often resort to games to keep control of their life but also to regain some control over yours'. Children may also become surprisingly good, not only to get your attention but as a way of protecting and looking after you. Adolescents may rebel and resort to forms of behaviour that can be as destructive to them as they are disturbing to you. Overwhelming grief is nearly always behind these angry verbal or behavioural outbursts. As hard as it may be, allowing them to express these emotions even when they are directed at you is more beneficial than any reprimand. This is painful stuff and professional guidance is often required to help you navigate this uphill path (See also Chapter 12).

These scenarios are hard to avoid as the repercussions of illness and death spread far beyond the visible horizon and may engulf many innocent people in their wake. The loss of what was once normal, the uncertainty and insecurity that follow, are all part of a child's grief and cannot be avoided. To the best of their ability, children need to understand what is happening to their sibling and why their own life and relationships have changed. This does not alter their grief for what is lost, but it may remove the sense of abandonment and guilt that invariably goes with it. It is not uncommon for children to wonder if they are to blame for whatever is happening or, alternatively, they may blame their sick sibling. Either scenario will sooner or later result in guilt.

There are no rules to follow but the siblings of a dying child need to understand and be understood. In keeping with what has been said about grief to date, let them ask the questions and if for any reason they cannot, ask them how they feel or how things have changed and take your cues from there. Young children may not understand when you ask how they feel. In that situation it is okay to ask if they feel sad. Give them plenty of time to think and reflect and to be as vulnerable as they are prepared to be. There can never be too many cuddles and kisses!

All that has just been said is also true, to a greater or lesser degree, when death involves some other family member. Grief associated with the death of a parent equals, and generally surpasses, that associated with the death of a sibling. The role the person played in the life of the child, the circumstances surrounding the loss and the age of the child are the most important factors that influence a child's grief. Death of a parent not only results in the loss of a very significant person but also the object of the child's love and affection. This results in ongoing and seemingly insurmountable changes that the child must contend with. Given the shock, disbelief, devastation and loss of control that accompanies such a tragedy, it is not surprising that the death of a parent can be more of a catastrophe for children than for adults, and that emotional, behavioural and social struggles often ensue.

The task for the surviving parent(s) is monumental as they struggle with their own grief while attempting to give emotional and physical support to the child (children) and keep the home together and the household running. As far as a child's grief is concerned the most important thing a surviving parent can do is to help their child mourn. This is very difficult for someone who is also grieving the loss of someone they love. Therese Rando, bereavement specialist and author of *How To Go On Living When Someone You Love Dies*, makes the following recommendations:

- Give affection and security.
- Look for ways to help your child express their emotions.
- Recognise that your child is also grieving the loss of a way of life, so keep things as 'normal' as possible.
- Encourage your child to talk with friends.
- Be aware your child will need times of solitude.

Research from the Harvard Bereavement Study in the United States has shown that allowing a grieving child to remain connected in some way to the dead parent can also be beneficial. This may be as simple as encouraging them to keep photos or memorabilia in their bedroom or by prompting them to talk about the deceased parent. Silence and trying to forget are clearly unhelpful. Those of you who wish to find out more about the effect of terminal illness on family life are directed to the Ockham's Razor programme, broadcast by the ABC on the 7th February 2010. In this recorded interview Dr Jane Turner, Senior Lecturer in Psychiatry at the University of Queensland, talks about her own and other research into the impact that parental cancer and subsequent death has on children. The programme link is: www.abc.net.au/ockhamsrazor/stories/2010.

Dr Averil Stedeford, a psychiatrist attached to several palliative care units in England, has some good advice on the way children can be prepared for the death of a parent. The most important considerations, she says, are the parents' own attitude to death, their openness with the children, and the amount of support children get from the extended family – the influence of grandparents is invaluable. The parents themselves often benefit from hearing how families in a similar position to theirs managed, and from confidence expressed by others in their ability to handle the situation well.

Therese Rando says, 'The main point and bottom line is very simple: Children do grieve. They need the help of adults to cope with major loss.'

Chapter 9

Care of the elderly

No one gets out of this world alive

WOODY ALLEN

Chapter 9

Care of the elderly

With more and more people living into their eighties and beyond, Australia, like most Western countries, has become an ageing society. Longevity, however, is not a privilege belonging to all. In Australia the notable exceptions are people of Aboriginal descent and those from poorer socio-economic groups. Life expectancy amongst these groups is 15 to 20 years less than average, and death results from illnesses that are related to living conditions and life style, and are therefore preventable.

The reason we have an ageing society is complex, but put simply it is because more and more people are living beyond the age of 65 years. The number of people over the age of 65 has doubled in the last forty years, and the fastest growing group is the 80-year-old and older population. This is unprecedented, and while it is good news for the present and coming generations it does have its down side. Ageing is often accompanied by chronic illness, increased risk of injury, limited mobility, social dislocation, death of a partner, friends and other family members, and a greater dependency on community services, and so the list goes on. Dementia is one of the scourges of ageing and it is estimated that 25 per cent of people who live to 85 years and beyond will have dementia.

If the number of people living longer is increasing, the number of older people dying must also be increasing. Many of these deaths occur in aged care facilities (previously known as nursing homes), but hospitals are the place where most will die. Overall, 90 per cent of the older age group will die in an institution. For this reason alone it is important that we examine how this group is cared for within our hospitals and other health care facilities.

The topics I will cover in this chapter are:

- the role of hospitals or aged care facilities in the care of those who are dying
- the commonest causes of death in the older age groups and the management of these illnesses. The illnesses include heart and lung disease, stroke, leukaemia, lymphoma and kidney failure. Cancer is not included as it has been fully covered in other chapters
- the special challenges faced when caring for the elderly person with dementia.

Dying in hospital

Hospital use is greatest amongst the elderly. This should come as no surprise considering the nature and number of illnesses that are common to this population. High blood pressure, diabetes mellitus, coronary artery disease, emphysema, strokes, arthritis, osteoporosis and circulation problems are just a few of the diseases that contribute to the deteriorating health of the aged. Rarely do these ailments appear in isolation. Evidence suggests the majority of the elderly population have chronic complex medical problems that not only impair quality of life but also increase dependence on medical services and necessitate frequent hospital admissions. Many of these admissions are for falls and accidents that result from limited mobility associated with the ageing process.

Statistics from the Australian Institute of Health and Welfare show that people aged 65 years and older are admitted to hospital more often than those below the age of 65, and that their length of stay is longer. Almost 90 per cent of the elderly are hospitalised in their last year of life and approximately 60 per cent die in hospital. Given these statistics it is reasonable to ask how the dying are cared for in hospitals.

It has been said that hospitals are not a good place to die. This statement is not a reflection on the level of care people receive within a hospital but on the nature of that care. Hospitals are places where people are admitted in the hope of making them better. The mindset that prevails, therefore, is one where lack of improvement, particularly if this leads to death, is considered a failure. So, even when death is seemingly inevitable, when all the signs suggest there is only one possible outcome, the medical profession tries harder and harder to overcome that which we all fear, namely death. It comes as no surprise then to know that 40 per cent of a person's health cost for the final year of life is spent in the last month of life. In other words, the sicker the person, the greater is the effort in trying to keep them alive. There are many studies from the United States and Australia that look at this in some detail. All of them show that hospital medicine rarely recognises death as an acceptable or inevitable end point and that the majority of people who die in hospital are receiving some form of active or potentially life-saving treatment at the time of their death. As Dr Michael Ashby, a professor of palliative medicine, said, the focus is less on dying and more on its prevention.

My purpose in exposing this is not to criticise what is done in hospital, or the people that work there, but only to point out that we (meaning all who work within the health care system) can do a little better when it comes to caring for the dying. There are ways we can ensure quality end-of-life care for those that die in hospital. Because the focus of this book is on carers, I will not talk about the steps hospitals can take, but about the things you can do to ensure the best quality care for a loved one who may be dying in hospital.

This is a complex matter, but the best place to start is to contemplate what constitute a so-called *good death*. The term 'a good death' may seem something of a oxymoron, but what I am really hoping to tease out are the things that may be important for someone who is dying and for those that are left to grieve. These are starting points for you and your family to consider when you are trying to ensure the best possible care for your dying loved one.

The following twelve principles of a good death are the brainchild of The Age Health and Care Study Group from the United Kingdom and were first published in *The Future of Health and Care of Older People* in 1999. I discovered them in a *British Medical Journal* the following year. While they were not written specifically for the hospital scene, they apply as much to hospitals as to any other place of death. I have found them to be useful in my work as a palliative care doctor and hope you, too, see their worth. The twelve principles are:

1. to know when death is coming, and to understand what can be expected
2. to be able to retain control of what happens
3. to be afforded dignity and privacy
4. to have control over pain relief and other symptoms
5. to have choice and control over where death occurs
6. to have access to information and expertise of whatever kind is necessary
7. to have access to any spiritual or emotional support required
8. to have access to palliative care
9. to have control over who is present and who shares the end
10. to be able to issue advance directives which ensure wishes are respected
11. to have time to say goodbye, and control over other aspects of timing
12. to be able to leave when it is time to go, and not to have life prolonged pointlessly.

If your loved one is in hospital and you think or are told he/she could be dying, I would recommend that you seek the services of the following people to help implement any or all of the above principles:

- a social worker
- the palliative care team
- the pastoral care team.

Representatives from one or all of these disciplines will not only meet with you, they will also provide information you and your loved one may require to make appropriate care choices around this time. They will also liaise closely with other specialists to ensure your loved one's wishes are carried through. Apart from this they can and will, if necessary, act as advocates and will help you to negotiate many of the challenges that confront you. Although hospitals struggle with the thought that death is natural and inevitable they have, in recent years, recognised the importance of providing appropriate end-of-life care and most large hospitals now have a palliative care team who can be called upon when required. They have also instituted end-of-life pathways to ensure patients who are dying receive the best and most appropriate care and that their family is kept informed and supported throughout the course of the illness.

As a relative or friend it is hard for you to know if and when your loved one is dying, yet, in the absence of an advance care directive (see below), you are the one who will be asked to decide about the continuation or withdrawal of treatment. You will be guided by the medical team, but the final decision will always be yours. Irrespective of the circumstances, the decision to withdraw treatment and recognise the inevitability of death is always painful – it will seem like giving up and you may feel as if you have failed your loved one.

The loss of someone you love is painful but the decision to stop treatment does not mean you are causing their death. Death, in the circumstances we are talking about, is inevitable. A decision to cease treatment is not the equivalent of a 'death sentence' but an acknowledgement of the truth. It is painful yet necessary. It recognises the futility of ongoing treatment, gives you and your family time to prepare for the death, to grieve and to introduce rituals that honour and celebrate the life of the one who is dying.

Dying in an Aged care Facility (Nursing Home)

Nursing homes have often been referred to as 'God's waiting room'. I am not sure if this accurate or helpful, but the fact remains – a significant proportion of the aged population spends their last years in an aged care facility and almost 90 per cent of those that live there will die there.

When I first commenced medical practice 43 years ago, many elderly people were admitted to nursing homes because they had nowhere else to live or were unable to care for themselves. Times have changed and so too has the profile of nursing home residents. Many are extremely ill with cancer, dementia or other life-threatening illness, so much so that nursing homes are now de facto palliative care units. Not surprisingly, then, many of the residents have symptoms one would expect in a palliative care population, namely pain, shortness of breath, loss of appetite, nausea, delirium, fatigue and constipation. The management of these symptoms has been detailed in earlier chapters and what is said there applies equally to nursing home residents and palliative care patients.

Although the reasons for admission to a nursing home are many and varied, families of nursing home residents are invariably confronted with difficult decisions that may have life or death implications. They may, for example, be asked to make a choice about:

- the initiation of treatment for a potentially life-threatening illness
- the appropriateness of antibiotics for a newly acquired infection
- the need for supplementary or artificial feeding
- the withdrawal of treatment that can no longer be swallowed or which now seems inappropriate
- transfer to a hospital.

Even though most nursing home residents have multiple and complex medical problems that contributed to their admission, many have a good quality of life. They are, however, susceptible to any number of health issues and the risk of a life-threatening complication is always on the 'cards'. If decisions are left until a crisis occurs, the choice will, in most instances, be to intervene. In some instances this may turn out to be correct, but it could, just as easily be wrong. The important point is that nursing home residents are at risk of developing serious complications and decisions regarding treatment should, if circumstances allow, be made pre-emptively and by the residents themselves. The only way this can be ensured is through an advance care directive.

An advance care directive, sometimes called a 'living will', is defined by NSW Health as a document that details a person's future preferences for medical treatment in anticipation of a time when he/she is unable to express those preferences because of illness or injury. What this means is that the resident, while they are capable, has the final say in their treatment. If, however, they are incapable or unable to do this, the next of kin makes a decision based on the explicit or implicit wishes of the resident as expressed in the directive. In effect this spares family the burdensome task and onerous responsibility of making life and death choices, for all they are doing is carrying out their next of kin's wishes.

So if your loved one has not already completed an advance care directive I would urge you to discuss this with them and to then seek guidance from your local doctor on how best to complete the directive. Conversations about advance planning are never easy and in some instances they are avoided because of the fear of alarming the person concerned. Remember, we are not asking you to talk about death and dying, but about how best to care for someone if they become seriously ill and are unable to participate in their choice of treatment. It is planning for the future, a future that is uncertain only because of the age and health of the resident.

The legislation concerning advance care directives is different in each state and territory. If, however, the directive is completed voluntarily by someone of sound mind, is witnessed and is relatively current, it is recognised under common law and its directives must be complied with, provided they are reasonable and within the law. An advance care directive completed in one state is valid in other Australian states and territories.

Dementia

If there is one thing people fear more than cancer it would have to be dementia. Dementia not only takes away one's life but also one's personality, dignity, independence, and way of life. From an outsider's point of view it slowly destroys a person's body, mind and soul and leaves only the skeletal remains of the individual they once knew. In its more advanced stages, people with dementia require a level of care that is hard to provide within the home. Most, therefore, require high level care within special dementia units attached to nursing homes.

Dementia is one of the prices we, as a society, pay for living longer. It is, for the most part, a disease of old age. Australian Health and Welfare statistics tell us that 5 per cent of people between 65 and 84 years have dementia, but this figure rises to almost 25 per cent for those aged 85 years and above.

The most common cause of dementia is Alzheimer's disease. Despite years of research the exact cause of Alzheimer's disease remains unknown. There are, however, numerous other causes including cerebro-vascular-disease (mini strokes), alcohol, brain injury, Parkinson's disease and other degenerative diseases of the brain. Progressive loss of memory is one of the earliest signs of dementia. This is slow and insidious and often overlooked until other behavioural or emotional changes appear. These changes include incontinence of urine, getting lost, missing appointments, domestic accidents, failure to recognise family or friends, apathy, anxiety and paranoia. This complex of symptoms and behavioual changes is sufficient to distinguish benign memory disturbance of old age from dementia.

Although there are now drugs that purport to slow the progression of

Alzheimer's disease there is no know cure, and most that develop this disease die in a matter of years from one of many sequelae including infection, poor nutrition or fractures (resulting from falls).

If your loved one has dementia there are several cross-roads you will have to negotiate during the course of their illness. The most important ones are:

- maintenance of meaningful social contact
- maintenance of nutrition
- pain control
- treatment of life-threatening complications.

Maintenance of meaningful social contact. Relatives of a person with dementia often say there is little value in visiting their demented relative. They feel frustrated and occasionally angry at the person's inability to communicate and conclude the visit does not benefit them or their sick relative. They not only stop their own visits but also those of other family members, including grandchildren. This is sad for all concerned, and particularly the children. From my experience children are more comfortable than adults in relating to a person with dementia and often maintain connections that adults struggle to make.

What we tend to forget is that people with dementia are, first and foremost, people. In the words of the now deceased British psychologist, Tom Kitwood, the *Who* (the person) must take precedence over the *What* (the Alzheimer's patient). In practice this means we should respect and relate to people with this illness in whatever way we can and not be sidetracked by seeing them as a case of Alzheimer's disease. In some strange and mysterious way, that W*ho* is there and at times this may be evident in what they say or do. A word, a smile of recognition or a tear often betrays the image we form of the person before us. This connection often comes when an emotional cord is struck through music, a photo, a smile, laughter, touch or simply by your silent presence. This is not surprising as the emotional memory is more hard wired and is therefore less susceptible than ordinary memory and cognition to the ravages of Alzheimer's disease.

This explains why people with advanced dementia can sing or hum along to familiar tunes and laugh or cry but cannot remember their name or respond to a simple question. One carer said, 'In many ways the deepest revelation of the Alzheimer journey is that it is a kind of passage from the mind into the heart'.

People with Alzheimer's struggle with words but their understanding and appreciation of things at a feeling level persist well into the disease. So when it comes to communication, it is us and our usual pattern of relating that need to change. Learning to communicate in ways other than words is one of the challenges you face in caring for someone with dementia, but the greater challenge is to overcome the common perception that people with dementia are 'not there'. They may be lost, but your task is to not find them – given time and sufficient emotional cues, they will sometimes find you.

Nutrition. Many people with dementia have difficulty with eating and on rare occasions will refuse food altogether. Weight loss is therefore very common and the question ultimately arises as to whether these people would benefit from nutritional supplements or some form of artificial feeding via a tube into the stomach (a PEG tube; see Chapter 4 and 5 for details).

There has, in recent years, been a tendency to resort to artificial feeding, particularly in the United States, where 25 per cent of those with dementia are fed via a PEG tube. Australia has been much slower in adopting this practice and not without good reason, for the evidence now suggests that PEG feeding is no better than taking food by mouth. The person's weight may remain stable or increase a little but complications associated with PEG feeding are high. Most importantly, the quality of life does not improve nor do people with PEG feeding live longer than those without.

While you may be alarmed by your relative's failure to eat and their subsequent weight loss, rest assured, if this is happening, he/she will not feel hungry and will not die of starvation. The situation is very similar to that of cancer in that the failure to eat and the resulting weight loss are a consequence of the disease and attempts to reverse the weight loss is doomed to fail while the disease remains unchecked. So do not attempt to make your loved one eat; give them what they want, when they want it. Do not make food and its consumption your priority and do not feel guilty if they do not eat. This is not something you can have any influence over. Being there with them is more important and more nourishing to their spirit.

Pain is as common a problem in people with dementia as it is with any elderly person or nursing home resident. The pain may be related to a pre-existing disease such as arthritis or may be secondary to an unrecognised infection or to muscle stiffness and soreness from immobility. If pain medication was required beforehand it should be continued, and in most instances, continued until they die.

Rarely do people with dementia complain of pain. Quite often it is suspected only because of non-verbal cues such as grimacing or shouting whenever they are touched or moved. This is particularly true if the behavioural change is new and there are no other obvious explanations. Of course, it is hard to know if the behavioural change is due to pain and sometimes a trial of medication is the only way to find out. The elderly are sensitive to most medications, including pain relievers, so if an analgesic is commenced, do not be surprised if the doctor starts with a small dose or tries some non-drug means of controlling the pain before resorting to an analgesic. If an analgesic is commenced, a Norspan® patch is often the treatment of choice because of its gentler and longer duration of action, and because it does not have to be swallowed.

Initiation and withdrawal of treatment. For most elderly people, particularly those with dementia, there comes a time when choices have to made about treatment. This may be about commencing treatment, often an antibiotic for an infection or, alternatively, about withdrawing treatment because the person is too unwell or is unable to swallow. In most instances the decision is clear cut but there are times when you will be uncertain and need guidance. Your doctor or nurse will give you all the necessary information to help you make an informed decision, but an advance care directive, if completed and current, will be your best guide.

As your loved one's health deteriorates, many of the medications previously considered important will no longer be necessary and may even cause problems if continued. This includes medication for blood pressure, heart trouble, diabetes mellitus, depression, Parkinson's disease et cetera. I find these medications, if continued into the later stages of a life-threatening illness (including dementia, now the fourth commonest cause of death in Australia), will only add to the burden of symptoms already being experienced. At this stage in a person's life the fewer tablets they have to take the better – so often, those that can will express relief at not having to swallow so many pills!

From my experience the greatest difficulty is not with stopping treatment but in not commencing treatment for an infection. Chest and urinary infections are common in people dying of dementia and to not start treatment is often felt to be a death sentence. The decision for or against antibiotics does, of course, depend on the circumstances and so it is not possible to make a blanket statement that covers all eventualities. All I wish to point out is that there may come a time when the infection is part and parcel of the dying process and treatment of the infection will not prevent death but will only prolong the dying. In these instances infection can be seen as a painless end to a person's suffering.

Hospital transfer. Whether you are caring for your loved one at home or if they are in a nursing home there are times when admission to a nearby hospital or hospice is entertained. Occasionally this may be necessary, but in the majority of instances hospital or hospice transfer is unlikely to benefit your loved one. This is particularly true if the problem is an infection, pain (or other symptoms) and minor trauma. In most instances these can be treated at home or in a nursing home. More importantly, keeping the person in a familiar environment avoids the distress and disorientation that follows when their sensory environment is changed.

The same rationale applies for when your loved one is dying. The level of resources available at home or within a nursing home is such that transfer to a hospice or hospital is rarely necessary. Pain and symptom control can, more often than not, be managed by your doctor and the nurses. If required a local palliative care specialist can be called in to advise if there is a difficult management issue. Carer exhaustion reaches its zenith at this time and is one of the few genuine reasons to consider transfer from home to hospice. This not only gives you much needed respite, but also frees you to be there with them as their loving spouse, partner or relative rather than the de facto nurse and doctor. The quality of your presence is most important around the time of your loved one's death and if this is dependent on you relinquishing your carer role, so be it.

Causes of death in the elderly

Along with cancer and dementia, the commonest causes of death in Australia are heart disease, strokes and emphysema.

Stroke is probably the commonest cause of death in the older age group and results from a sudden reduction or cessation of blood flow to a critical part of the brain. The commonest area affected is that part of the brain responsible for movement, so the cardinal feature of a stroke is paralysis or weakness on the opposite side of the body. Difficulty with speaking is only a problem if the dominant side of the brain is affected (left side of the brain for right-handed people and vice versa).

Strokes may result from a clot (also called a thrombosis) blocking one of the major arteries of the brain, a haemorrhage or rupture of a major blood vessel, or an embolus. With the latter, a small clot forms in the heart or a blood vessel outside of the brain, breaks off and travels within the circulation until it lodges in a smaller artery. In the case of an embolic stroke the embolus lodges in a small artery in the brain.

Apart from paralysis, strokes can result in loss of consciousness or coma, difficulty with swallowing, and pneumonia. The chance of survival diminishes with any of these complications and is most unlikely if all three are present. The degree of recovery following a stroke depends on the extent of the underlying brain damage. The damage is greatest with thrombosis and slight with embolus, and so recovery is more likely with the latter. Rehabilitation is a necessary part of the recovery process and can last for weeks or years depending on the extent of the stroke and the resulting paralysis.

Apart from paralysis, it is not uncommon to have one or more of the following complicate the recovery period: pain, confusion, disorientation, difficulty with swallowing, musculo-skeletal problems, falls, fractures, spasticity, pressure areas, and chest and urinary infections. The prevention and management of each of these is beyond the scope of this book but further information can be obtained from your local doctor or the rehabilitation service involved in your loved one's care.

There are many difficult decisions you may be asked to make, particularly in the early phase of your loved one's stroke. These include the question of transfer to an intensive care unit, artificial ventilation, artificial feeding, new and innovative ways of treating the stroke and finally the issue of antibiotics for a chest or urinary infection. Each of these is almost too overwhelming to consider, particularly as the decisions need to be made in the first hours to days after the stroke. My recommendation is that you get as much information as you can from the treating specialist and then discuss the matter fully with all family members, utilising the services of the hospital social worker or pastoral care worker. Your final decision should always be guided by a valid and current advance care directive, but failing that, you should ask yourself, what would your loved one choose in this situation?

The question of antibiotics, artificial feeding, initiation and withdrawal of treatment has already been addressed in this and other chapters. Pain management follows the principles outlined in Chapter 3 and information on confusion (delirium), management of pressure areas and the treatment of chest and urinary infections can be found in Chapter 4. It is not uncommon for palliative care to be involved in the management of any or all of these problems and with end-of-life care, if and when death seems inevitable. The issue of comfort and care around the end of life is just as important following a stroke as it is with cancer.

Heart disease remains the commonest cause of death in the Western world, but accounts for fewer deaths amongst the elderly than do strokes. The commonest heart conditions are angina and a heart attack (coronary occlusion). The former is a result of marked narrowing of one or more coronary arteries. Heart attack, on the other hand, is due to a complete blockage of one coronary artery. Only the latter results in damage to the heart, but both are potentially fatal at their initial presentation and at any time thereafter. With prolonged or severe coronary artery disease, heart muscle can be so starved of oxygen that it fails to function normally and this leads to what is called *congestive heart failure*. As the name suggests, fluid builds up in the body, leading to swelling of the legs and increasing breathlessness secondary to congestion of the lungs. Numerous medications are now available for the treatment of angina and congestive failure, and a reasonable quality of life can be maintained for months to years depending on the severity of the underlying disease

Palliative care involvement usually comes late in the course of heart disease, usually when pain and breathlessness is troublesome and unresponsive to the usual medication. The management of each of these symptoms has been detailed in Chapters 3 and 4 and what is recommended there for pain and breathlessness is as valid for late stage coronary artery disease and congestive heart failure as it is for cancer.

Emphysema is a chronic lung condition usually, but not always a result of smoking. Irreversible damage to the minute air sacs in the lungs interferes with the gas exchange that normally takes place. This results in breathlessness, which in its severest form can limit movement to a just a few paces. Cough and wheezing are also prominent features of this disease.

Palliative care is often called upon to assist in managing the breathlessness, and the principles involved are no different to that outlined in Chapter 4. The only point that needs to be emphasised is that morphine is a very important and almost an essential part of the medical management. I stress this only because there is a long-held myth that morphine is contraindicated and potentially dangerous in people with emphysema or other forms of chronic lung disease. The evidence is now quite clear that morphine, in appropriate doses, improves breathing and the quality of life of people with emphysema. The dose required is often smaller than that for pain and, as with pain, the morphine is given regularly rather than intermittently, with breakthrough doses for severe exacerbations of breathlessness.

If not introduced earlier in the course of this condition, morphine is certainly indicated in its final stages. Either alone or in combination with a mild sedative it can ease the distress of not getting enough breath that would otherwise characterise the time of dying. People living with emphysema often tell me they're not as afraid of death as they are of the way they will die. What they fear is 'suffocation'. The judicious use of morphine and other medications at the time of their dying should ensure this never happens.

Kidney or 'renal' failure is the tenth commonest cause of death in Australia but is the commonest amongst Aborigines. Renal failure is rife amongst this and Indigenous groups in other countries because of the extremely high incidence of diabetes mellitus and high blood pressure within these populations.

The early phase of treatment aims to control these diseases. Medications and strict adherence to a special diet are also essential at this time. As the renal failure worsens, the kidneys are unable to eliminate all the body's waste products and survival depends on a machine that, in effect, takes the place of the kidneys. This process of removing excess water and toxic waste products from the blood of a person with renal failure is called *dialysis*. This procedure is carried out two to three times a week and unless the person is one of the few lucky ones to receive a renal transplant, dialysis continues for the remainder of their life. For some, particularly the aged or those burdened with other illnesses, there comes a time when on-going dialysis becomes overly burdensome. These people are counselled about their options, one of which is terminating dialysis which, in most cases, leads to death in a matter of days or weeks.

Palliative care practitioners often become involved at this point. Some of their tasks include counselling the patient and his/her family, palliating troublesome symptoms and, finally, ensuring a peaceful death. Some of the symptoms that may appear around this time, or before, include breathlessness, nausea, vomiting, hiccups, drowsiness, confusion, itch and pain. They are all treated along the lines outlined in Chapters 3 and 4, but with special care taken in the choice and dose of medication. In the case of pain or breathlessness, morphine is often contraindicated as the risk of side effects is high in those with renal failure. For this reason, fentanyl or methadone is preferred.

Leukaemia and lymphoma are forms of cancer that involve the blood and lymph tissue respectively. Neither is confined to the elderly, but both are common to that age bracket. Once considered incurable, there are now various treatment modalities, including chemotherapy, radiotherapy and transfusion that prolong survival and not infrequently result in cure.

Either the illness itself or its treatment can result in symptoms, many of which respond to palliative measures. These symptoms include pain, breathlessness, fatigue, bleeding or bruising tendencies, loss of appetite, weight loss, nausea and vomiting.

Fatigue may be secondary to anaemia and often improves with a blood transfusion. Bleeding and bruising results from a low platelet count – platelets are manufactured in the bone marrow and are often reduced in number as a result of the illness or its treatment. This bleeding tendency is temporarily improved by platelet transfusions.

The treatment of leukaemia and lymphoma often continues until well into the palliative phase of the illness and is ceased only when the disadvantages of treatment, namely the side effects, outweigh the benefits. At this point treatment becomes purely palliative, with symptom management and ultimately end-of-life care becoming the major foci of attention.

Perhaps the hardest decision that confronts all people with a life-threatening illness is when to cease active treatment. This is particularly true for leukaemia and lymphoma and involves decisions not only around the usefulness of chemotherapy but also regarding the value of on-going transfusions. It is the latter that causes most angst and for that reason transfusion is often continued late into the course of the illness and is only withdrawn when it clearly offers no benefits or when death is near.

Dying of 'old age'

A bird sings louder as you grow older

ROSE CHERNIN

The somewhat misleading phrase – 'dying of old age' – puts 'old age' in the same category as other life-threatening illness. It is a sad and erroneous take on old age, for old age itself is not a terminal disease. Certainly there are biological changes that result in loss of strength, agility and mobility. The chance of acquiring diseases that are truly life-threatening also increases. Life is finite and while a select few survive to 85 years and beyond, what kills them is not their age but the illnesses or accidents they acquire along the way. Age does not appear in the 'commonest causes of death' list nor is it recognised as a cause of death by the Registry of Births, Deaths and Marriages. Consequently it never appears on a death certificate as a cause of death.

Because the likelihood of death increases as we get older, aging is not only a time to enjoy and savour but it is also a time to prepare for our death. This may sound a little morbid, but death is inevitable. As Woody Allen says, 'No one gets out of this world alive'. While we know this to be true very few of us in the Western world prepare for death. The reasons are many and varied but because we do not prepare for it, we are often caught unawares and fear it, as Philippe Ariés said, as a child fears the dark. Preparing for death is not as morbid as it sounds. It not only involves practical matters such as wills and advance care directives; it also means completing all our unfinished business. Sometimes this business may be materialistic, such as visiting people or places, or it may be more spiritual, as in trying to be a better person. Indian culture has seen the value of preparing for death and has accordingly divided life into four stages or *ashramas*:

1. **Brahmacarya or the formative years** – when we grow and mature
2. **Garhasthya or the materialist years** – when we acquire wealth and status
3. **Vanarprasthya or the stable years** – when we start to reduce our wants and needs
4. **Sannyasa or the years of wisdom** – when we prepare for our death.

We in the Western world have adopted the first two stages but somehow have become stuck in the materialistic stage. Maybe it is time to move on, but first we need to see the value in preparing for death. For me the reason can be found in the words of Archbishop Desmond Tutu, 'unless you look the beast in the eye you will find that it returns to hold you hostage'. Death deserves respect and, like any significant life event, we fare better if we prepare adequately for it.

Chapter 10

Motor Neuron Disease

'Ageing is just not decay. . . . It's growth.
It's more than the negative that you're going to die,
it's also the positive that you understand
you're going to die, and that you live a better life
because of it.'

MORRIE SCHWARTZ
Tuesdays with Morrie by Mitch Albom

Chapter 10

Motor Neuron Disease

T*uesdays with Morrie* has become one of the 'must read' books for anyone interested in the subject of motor neuron disease (MND). It is the true story of Morrie Schwartz, an ageing university professor, who, while dying of the disease, gives a 'final class' to a previous student and author of the book, Mitch Albom, on how to live. It is a beautifully crafted story that shows there is another side to the devastation that accompanies any life-threatening illnesses, including MND.

These days, *cancer* is the disease we all fear and hope never to get. The very mention of the word conjures up thoughts of pain, suffering and an untimely death. If given a choice, almost everyone would prefer any other illness rather than suffer the ravages of cancer. There are, however, several lesser-known illnesses that can be just as devastating and unattractive. One of these is motor neuron disease. Like cancer, it is a wasting disease that gradually (sometimes rapidly) erodes a person's independence as it relentlessly pursues its course towards death. Unlike cancer, there is no recognised treatment or hope for remission, let alone cure. The diagnosis of MND is as much a death sentence as is cancer and presents the carer and the cared for with many challenges. Some of these challenges are similar to those with cancer, but many are specific to MND, and it is for this reason that a special chapter has been devoted to it.

The cause of motor neuron disease is unknown. It affects adults of all age groups and results in progressive weakness and wasting of the muscles of the body, often starting in the small muscles of the hand. From there it spreads to involve all muscles of the upper and lower limbs. The muscles concerned with speech and swallowing are often affected later in the disease but can, in some instances, be involved from the outset. Occasionally the weakness starts in the legs, and then the rate of disease progression is often slower.

The distribution of the weakness and the rate of progression vary considerably, but all those with MND are ultimately confined to a wheel chair and have difficulty with speech and swallowing. Muscle cramps are frequent and pain from stiffness and spasticity often requires treatment with strong analgesics such as morphine. Sensation is always preserved, as is bowel and bladder function. Both, however, may be compromised by generalised weakness – so much so that a urinary catheter and assistance with toileting is almost always required at some later stage. As the disease progresses, the major issues that confront the person with MND are as follows:

Loss of independence. Ultimately assistance is required for all activities of daily living, such as toileting, showering, feeding and mobility. Initially you, the carer, may be able to provide all the necessary assistance. In time, additional help will, almost certainly, be required and this may come from family, friends or community services. Various home aids, including an ordinary and an electric wheelchair, will also be necessary. Advice about home aids and where they can be obtained is available through your community nurse, doctor or the MND Association (see Appendix)

Difficulty with swallowing. Initially, this problem may require only minor modifications to the diet and the way food is presented. As the difficulty progresses, a change to soft or pureed foods will become essential, but even then the effort and time taken to consume blended food will often result in an inadequate caloric intake, aggravating the problem of weight loss secondary to muscle wasting. You may be surprised to find that your loved one will have more difficulty swallowing fluids than solids. This is because fluids pass from the mouth to the swallowing tube faster than solids and in the face of muscle weakness this cannot be controlled adequately, and can result in small amounts of the liquid entering the breathing tubes. This leads to coughing and an increased risk of chest infections. For this reason care should be taken with liquids and nurses may recommend thickening agents to lessen the risk of inhalation.

Weight loss is inevitable with MND. It is not a major concern unless the loss is dramatic or the oral intake falls well below what would be considered 'normal' for the situation. In either of these situations, or when swallowing (food or fluids) results in coughing, some form of artificial feeding, usually through a PEG tube, needs to be considered. In fact the question of artificial feeding is best raised with your doctor well beforehand. This will allow for full and open discussion and for an informed rather than a rushed decision. If a PEG tube is to be inserted, this is usually done well before any of the above problems develop. More information on PEG tubes is provided in Chapter 4.

Chest infections. Chest infections secondary to the inhalation of fluids are one of the commonest problems associated with MND. A PEG tube reduces but does not eliminate this risk altogether, as difficulty in swallowing saliva can also predispose to chest infections. There are ways of reducing this risk and your community nurse can outline these. Medications are also used to reduce the volume of saliva and the amount of associated drooling – the source of much embarrassment for your loved one. These medications are moderately helpful and your doctor can provide further information on what is available, their benefits and their side effects.

The risk of chest infection also increases as coughing becomes less effective. We all make bronchial secretions, but our body automatically clears them throughout the day and night. When this clearing mechanism is impaired, as it is with MND, secretions will pool, increasing the risk of infection. Regular repositioning and the occasional use of antibiotics to prevent or treat infections are then recommended.

Communication. Difficulties with speech parallel the weakness in other muscles – the greater the weakness elsewhere, the harder it is for the person with MND to talk and be understood. This is a frustrating experience for you the carer as well as for your loved one. Various aids are available, and information about these is available through your state MND Association. Time, patience and intuition are, however, the keys to communication, irrespective of what aids you may or may not use.

Pain. Pain may be surprisingly severe and strong analgesics such as morphine are often prescribed. The pain may be related to muscle stiffness and spasticity or arise from a pre-existing problem such as arthritis or sciatica. In situations such as these, doctors may be reluctant to prescribe morphine and patients are equally loathe to accept it. This may be because of a fear about the use of morphine or a belief that morphine is only used for cancer or when someone is dying. Neither is true. Morphine is a safe and valuable means of improving physical comfort in those with MND and should be used earlier rather than later in the course of the disease.

I would add one word of caution: morphine and other strong analgesics are constipating and this can aggravate the difficulty most people with MND have in emptying their bowels. For this reason laxatives are almost always prescribed when an analgesic is commenced. In fact, laxatives are often required for all people with MND because of their inability to strain.

Difficulty with breathing. Just as all other muscle groups become weak, so too do the muscles of respiration. Difficulty with breathing is, however, a relatively late complication as the diaphragm, an important muscle of respiration, is not as severely affected as the muscles of the chest and can continue to do the job for some time after the chest and accessory neck muscles have failed.

When shortness of breath appears, home oxygen is beneficial (see Chapter 4 for more information on oxygen). In some cases this may not be adequate to relieve breathlessness, and for these people assisted ventilation via a mask is usually required. Assisted ventilation (within the home) is a relatively non-invasive procedure and is something you, the carer, or your loved one can manage quite easily. The need for this form of ventilation and the choice of apparatus, however, must be evaluated carefully. For this reason a neurologist, a respiratory or rehabilitation specialist is often consulted.

The place of assisted ventilation in an intensive care unit utilising a 'respirator' is a different matter altogether. A decision about this form of intervention arises for one of two reasons:

- to assist respiration while someone is receiving antibiotic treatment for a chest infection. Generally, ventilation in this situation is only considered useful if the person had a good quality of life before the infection and the likelihood of them returning to that state after treatment is high
- to support respiration towards the end of life.

Both of these scenarios raise complex social, medical and philosophical issues and are best discussed well before the need for ventilation arises. This should be done with the most senior doctor involved in the case, and if possible with relevant family members, the general practitioner and community nurse also present. The decision on ventilation, other forms of intervention and the nature of care at the end of life should then be documented in an Advance Care Plan and copies placed in the medical and nursing file. For more information on Advance Care Plans (Directives) see Chapter 9.

Depression. This is a not unexpected complication of MND. The gradual loss of independence, the inability to adequately communicate and the fear of choking or suffocating all contribute to a sense of despair and foreboding. For most people burdened with a life-threatening illness it is possible to defuse some of their angst and anxiety by allowing them to talk about their fears. The ability to do this becomes increasingly difficult with MND and reaches its zenith when the need to communicate is greatest. So what can be done?

There is no simple or glib answer to this dilemma. Hopefully all that needed to be said will have been said before this time, but even then fears resurface and need to be dealt with in some way. You can often tell or intuit when your loved one is down and more in need of your company. If you sense this, trust your intuition and sit with them, hold their hand and be fully present to their needs. They may not speak but their body language is powerful enough to deliver a message. Show that you care and love them, and offer whatever comfort or reassurance you think they need. If they have previously spoken about their fears or concerns, reassure them as often as you think necessary – redundancy is never a problem.

The doctor and community nurse have a very special part to play in all of this. They can fill in many of the gaps that are often a major source of concern, both for you and your loved one – they can talk about the unknown and what can be done to ensure a death that meets your loved one's needs and deals with his/her fears. Anti-depressants are sometimes indicated, but they are always additional to rather than a substitute for love, a comforting presence and meticulous planning of care.

You may think discussing such things as preparation for death and the prevention of suffocation and choking would be frightening for your loved one. My experience has been quite the opposite. All of my patients (not only those with MND) are relieved when the matter of death and dying is brought out into the open. It gives them the opportunity to talk about their fears, to hear what can be done to ensure a peaceful death, and then to negotiate a care plan with the doctor, nurse and family. Such a discussion becomes the basis for an Advance Care Plan that not only lets the doctor know how the person wishes to be cared for at the end of life, but also relieves the family of difficult decisions that might otherwise fall into their lap.

Good palliative care cannot alleviate the despair that goes with dying, nor should it try to, for this is a normal response to a life-threatening situation. Dying is not a problem that can be solved, but it invokes emotions that need to be expressed over and over again – as often as is necessary. Your task as a carer is to hear (or sense) thc pain that is being expressed and to show that you 'hear' the message they are giving – you do this with tears, a cuddle, a kiss and, if necessary, words of comfort.

What message can we take from all of this? Morrie Schwartz has the answer and it comes in two parts. When asked for his final words he said, 'Be compassionate' – that is his advice to those who care for the dying. In reference to his own illness (MND) he says, 'It'll get my body. It will not get my spirit'. Surely that is a message all of us – both the living and the dying – need to ponder.

Chapter 11

The inner journey

People die the way they have lived.

ANON

Chapter 11

The inner journey

Each of us is a unique and special person. Our personality is the visible manifestation of a complex mix of conscious, subconscious and unconscious forces that have been moulded together over the years by life's experiences, and by our personal, cultural, religious and spiritual beliefs. Our personality is the part of us that others get to know and like or dislike. The perception of who we really are is anything but clear to ourselves, let alone to others. This is not only because of the subtle effects of the 'invisible' unconscious but also because we, for a number of reasons, only reveal those parts of ourselves we are happy for others to know. The impression other people form is equally distorted by the spectacles through which they view us 'as they fail to see because of the pictures they paint on the glass' (Anon).

Rarely do we reveal that which is precious, singularly important or too painful to talk about. Sometimes, these matters are so deeply buried they are not even accessible to the conscious mind, but nonetheless they exist. The time of our death is one of the few occasions when deep or concealed parts of us can rise to the surface and influence the way we feel and behave. This can result in familiar but somewhat exaggerated behaviour, or behaviour that is quite out of character. The way we conduct ourselves may also be the product of an internal conflict where we struggle with ambivalence – a decision about revealing or concealing something of importance.

Reconciling such a difference is always liberating, particularly for those confronted by death. I do not wish to imply that every dying person has a skeleton in the cupboard or that the skeleton, if it exists, needs to be exposed. Significant issues, however, do arise and, when they do, it is important to allow a person to talk rather than for us to reassure or to dismiss the problem as unimportant. Being fully present and listening with an open heart and a closed mouth is all that is required; any form of disclosure could be cathartic and healing in its own right.

If a dying person starts to reveal their innermost secrets, you may feel inadequate to deal with their and your emotions. This is not an abnormal response. If it should happen, take a deep breath, cast aside (as best you can) your own fears and anxieties and trust yourself and the occasion. The dying person is speaking to you as their spouse, partner or friend. They are not expecting you to solve their problem, offer reassurance or venture forth with some hastily formed advice. Be reassured by the knowledge the dying person has chosen you to receive something of importance. It is a real gift and you can repay that gift with your time and undivided attention

The inner journey a dying person makes is as unique to them as their personality. The adage that people die the way they have lived is a piece of wisdom that helps us understand their journey and the many twists and turns it may take. If someone has been angry throughout life, don't be surprised if they are angry around the time of their death. Similarly, someone who has always cared for others may be more concerned about the welfare of the family than their own predicament. So, the more you get to know someone in life, the more you will understand them, their needs, wants and fears as they approach death. I learnt this lesson very early in my palliative care career and, as is often the case, my teacher was one of my patients. His name was Sam.

Sam was an elderly man who had reluctantly agreed to his landlady's request to enter the hospice. I will never forget our first meeting. He was unshaven and unclean and clearly uncomfortable with the spotless hospice surrounds. His hand was bandaged and as the dressing was removed he winced but never complained. Half of the hand had been eaten away by cancer and a large gaping hole was present where his armpit should have been. Knowing how painful this must have been, I was amazed that any person could let things get to this stage.

The cancer may have been beyond cure but I knew something could be done to ease Sam's pain. To my surprise he refused my offer of pain relief and the more I pressed the more adamant he was in refusing it. Finally, he said, 'I want to get out of here'. I had overstepped an invisible boundary. He insisted on leaving, but as it was then late in the day he agreed to delay his departure until the next morning, on the proviso there would be no further mention of pain relief. I breathed a sigh of relief and left, wondering what had gone wrong.

I rang the landlady to inform her of Sam's decision. She was not surprised and told me all she knew about him. He had spent all but the last few months of his life as a vagrant, sleeping outdoors, usually on park benches. He was a loner, his own master and never once sought or received help. I immediately understood why he was so uncomfortable with me, my plans for pain relief, and the surrounds he had unhappily found himself in.

I entered Sam's room the next morning, half expecting him to have vanished overnight. He was still there, propped up in bed, picking over breakfast with his one good hand. I apologised for yesterday's events and attempted to say goodbye. Sam said, 'I'm

> *still going, but I need my trousers cleaned.' He pointed to the drawer and sure enough the trousers were dirty, and I doubted if they had ever seen the inside of a washing machine. I said they might not be ready until tomorrow. 'That's okay', was Sam's reply. The next day I returned with the trousers. 'Thanks, but I might stay another night,' he said. And so he did. In fact, he stayed until he died some weeks later, having had no pain relief or any other medication throughout his whole stay.*

Sam taught me that people do, indeed, die the way they have lived. Their ability to do so, however, is often influenced by the circumstances they find themselves in and the level of discernment others show towards them. Sam had little of value in life other than life itself and the freedom to make his own decisions. The cancer was robbing him of the former and I, with my talk of pain relief, was robbing him of the latter. Once we got to know Sam, things changed and he was able to negotiate his illness and death in a manner of his choosing. Sam was anything but ordinary. Some may describe him as a misfit, but aren't we all? Being a misfit is nothing less than being unique and it is in our uniqueness that we discover dignity in life and in death. Much of our life is spent searching to understand ourselves (and others) and have others accept who we are. When our inner and outer world is in harmony with this aspiration, life flows and obstacles that once appeared insurmountable become unimportant. Such congruence is even more important with death and forms the basis of the poet Rainer Maria Rilke's exhortation 'Oh Lord, give each of us his own death'.

Things do not always work out as well as they did with Sam, or that's how it may seem on the surface. Many times I have left a dying person's side, feeling I had let them down in their time of need, only to hear at some later date how much they had benefited from the meeting. So often it is our own sense of inadequacy and helplessness that colours the end result. Dying people do not seek answers, only opportunities to express themselves. Never underestimate the power of two vulnerable people making meaningful contact. The words do not seem to matter, as care is not measured by what you say or do, but by how prepared you are to listen. By twisting a well-known adage, the social psychologist and author, Richard Kalish, tells us how this is done – 'Don't just do something, sit there.'

A final word of caution: the assertion that people die the way they have lived is generally true and a good indicator of how each of us might behave when death threatens. The danger is that this adage, if applied strictly, may see individuals labelled and packaged because of their past – other aspects of their nature that may rarely have surfaced but nonetheless exist could easily be overlooked because of a preconceived impression of who they are and what they need. When death threatens, change follows, so remain receptive at all times to the potential for change, not only with your loved one but also with yourself and others.

Grief

The process of change, the emotional ups and downs and the existential crises that occur when someone is dying are all part of a grief reaction. The Oxford Dictionary defines grief as a time of intense sorrow and sadness, and indeed it is, but it is much more than that. Grief is a whole-body experience and not just an emotional reaction that occurs in response to any form of loss. Neither is it a state, but rather a process that has been described by the author NW Clerk, as like a long valley where any bend reveals a totally new landscape. Grief is as unpredictable as life itself and the intensity of grief can vary enormously over any 24-hour period. The emotional component may be powerful and, if so, grief is easily recognised. If, however, grief takes on some of the other guises mentioned below it can be overlooked and in the case of a dying person, the symptoms may be wrongly attributed to the underlying illness.

In the context of dying, grief involves countless losses, not the least being the impending loss of one's own life. For you, the carer, relative or friend, it involves the loss of someone you love and loss of a way of life.

Whether it is the carer or the cared for, grief can manifest in any or all of the following ways:

- **Physical:** crying, loss of appetite, intense fatigue, constipation or diarrhoea, palpitations, sweating, difficulty with sleeping.
- **Mental:** apathy, forgetfulness, difficulty in concentrating.
- **Social:** withdrawal from friends and relatives; lack of interest in family and social activities.
- **Psychological:** a wide range of emotions of varying intensity and duration. These emotions often come in waves, reflecting the natural ebb and flow of despair and hope.
- **Existential:** questioning the meaning of life and death as well as religious and spiritual beliefs.
- **Paranormal:** unusual experiences are not uncommon when someone is confronted by the prospect of death. More is said about this in Chapter 6, 'States of Consciousness'.

Grief is a normal response to loss and, in the context of dying, may be profound and prolonged. Grief does not follow any pattern and the grieving process is as individual as a person's personality, so do not be alarmed if the descriptions that follow do not accurately describe what you see or experience. Grief arises from issues deep within and, just as a mirror reflects only superficial features, emotions and other visible features of grief are poor images of what is happening at a much deeper level.

Grief brings forth a whole raft of changes, not only for the one who is dying but also for family and close friends, and the resulting dynamics may be as distressing as the thought of death itself. One person I cared for recently said her greatest concern was not that she was dying but that her dying was tearing her family apart at a time when she longed for closeness and intimacy. While she struggled with the reality of approaching death, her family retreated from their own pain and sense of helplessness by distancing themselves physically and emotionally from her and the situation. There was no question about the love they felt for each other. Grief, however, had driven a wedge between them and rendered them strangers, lost to each other at the time of their greatest need. It is so easy to become lost in our own grief, and in struggling to keep our head above water we can become blinded to what is happening around us.

Dr Elisabeth Kübler-Ross was one of the first doctors to popularise the notion of grief in the context of dying. Current opinion suggests that her views may not be entirely accurate but they have contributed greatly to our understanding of the subject. She believed that grief occurred as a result of actual or anticipated loss. Grief, she said, is a whole-body experience and, while emotions take centre stage, the physical and mental effects and the ramifications of these on our life are as real and often more crippling. She described how grief unfolds and, while this was considered gospel for many years, her initial description has since been reviewed and reshaped. Grief does not necessarily progress in recognisable stages. It is unpredictable and as changeable as the weather but, like the weather, there are features and patterns we can recognise.

I will spend the remainder of this chapter talking about the different emotions that, together with other changes, combine to form the grief response. To describe each emotion separately, as I do, is artificial and potentially misleading – emotional states rarely exist as pure entities but are part of a kaleidoscope of feelings that have the potential to change with every turn in a person's life. It does, however, help us to appreciate the many 'primary' emotions that blend into the state of being we call grief.

What follows is based on observation and experience and is not a critical analysis of grief. It may not conform exactly to what the experts say, but my hope is that the recollections speak more about the human side of grief.

Fear

Fear does not stop death, it stops life.

ELISABETH KÜBLER-ROSS AND DAVID KESSLER
Life Lessons

Professor John Hinton in his classic text, *Dying*, lists many emotions that are aroused by the prospect of death, but says that fear is the commonest.

Fear characteristically varies in intensity throughout an illness. Some days it may be overwhelming and disabling, throwing a dark and lengthy shadow over life. At other times it may be almost non-existent. The reason for these fluctuations is not always clear; external factors may account for some of the changes but they may also be due to a deeply embedded survival mechanism where the psyche temporarily dissociates from what is really happening. Such dissociation is not uncommon and is a healthy coping mechanism, offering periods of respite for all concerned. Don't be surprised if fear reigns supreme one day and is gone the next.

A dying person's fear may have a specific focus – fear of death, fear of suffering, fear of separation from loved ones or of being alone at the time of death. It may also be existential, as the dying person questions long-held religious or philosophical beliefs or the meaning of their life. Mostly, it is a fear of the unknown.

Fear of death is often replaced by the fear of how the person will die, when it will happen and whether suffering will be part of that final act. The fear of death is never lost but death is seen as inevitable and accepted only because there is no escaping it. If there is no escape, they are more likely to focus attention on what is equally frightening but potentially within their control – the manner of their dying. In my experience, most people, particularly those with cancer, expect that they will die in pain. Those with lung cancer or emphysema are particularly concerned about the possibility of choking or suffocating. Sometimes, the dying person's fears are more akin to worries and relate to practical issues such as how their spouse/partner will manage or who will care for children. They may also be consumed by financial matters (more common with men), outstanding or unfinished household repairs, a car, a pet, their prized collection(s). Such concerns may seem trivial, but if they are raised they are important.

Whatever the fear or concern, no matter how significant or seemingly trivial, the opportunity for the dying person to talk and have someone listen is most therapeutic. A resolution may be possible, particularly if the problem is of a practical nature, but for all matters the opportunity to unburden can in itself be therapeutic. If the fear is overwhelming, persistent or hard to talk about, the assistance of a qualified counsellor may be necessary. Your general practitioner is the best person to assist you with these more complicated situations and if necessary they can direct you to a qualified counsellor. Referral to a counsellor or psychologist for grief is now included under Medicare and, depending on the counsellor's billing arrangements, this service is free or comes at a minimal cost.

Depression

Depression may not be something a dying person complains of, or is even aware of, but it is present in a large proportion of those who are dying. It is frequently overlooked, as the cardinal symptoms and signs of depression are sometimes indistinguishable from those of the underlying disease. Sadness, loss of appetite, lack of energy, loss of interest and difficulty sleeping are common to both depression and advanced disease and it can be difficult to know which is responsible. The simplest way of determining whether a person is depressed is to ask the obvious question – do you feel depressed?

The feeling of depression is a very normal response to the ravages of illness and the associated losses the person has suffered or is likely to suffer. The medical and social consequences of a terminal illness are 'painful' enough. Add to these the fear of the future, of suffering, of dying (or of not being able to die), concern about being a burden to the family and separation from all that a person loves, and it is not surprising that depression should occur. What is more surprising is that depression is not seen in everyone who is dying and that depression does not always turn into despair.

The difference between depression and despair (pathological depression) is subtle and one can imperceptibly merge into the other. While hard to make, the distinction is important. Despair is a much more serious form of depression, more disabling, associated with morbid thoughts of death and suicide, and frequently improves with antidepressant medication. There is no single feature that helps to distinguish one from the other, but the feelings of hopelessness, sadness and remorse are generally worse and talk of suicide more common in those with despair. The desire to die is not pathological and may in fact be normal in the circumstances. For that reason, a slow death or a belief that they cannot die may be more of a worry for some and the source of their despair.

In my experience, one of the main features of 'normal' depression and what distinguishes it from despair is the retention of some purpose or meaning in life despite all that is happening to them and around them. This purpose often revolves around family and long established relationships, the need to complete some unfinished business or the hope of surviving until some special person arrives or a significant milestone is achieved. This hope of survival not only gives the terminally ill a purpose in life; when attained it also gives them permission to die. So often we see people die a short time after their last wish has been fulfilled. Several of the stories that appear throughout the book illustrate this point.

One of the best ways you can care for someone who is down is to create a space where they feel safe and secure enough to talk. They may not use the word 'depression' and they may find it difficult to talk about how they feel, but they will be able to talk about their losses and other important things. Issues that may also arise include how the illness has affected their life and relationships, the things they are now unable to do and what death will rob them of. Be careful, however, not to make this a question and answer session. Allow the person to talk, let them direct the flow of the conversation, but listen carefully for cues and follow up with statements like, 'Tell me more about that'.

Such talk may be accompanied by tears. This can be disconcerting and the natural tendency is to change the subject in the belief it is too painful for the person to continue. Nothing is further from the truth. Tears suggest they are talking about issues that really matter and this ultimately brings healing. There is more reason for concern about the person who never cries.

In the face of tears it is best to remain silent and, if it seems appropriate, to make some physical contact to show that you are present to their pain. This contact must be appropriate – a hug if you are family, or a simple holding of the hand. Remember, the contact is not made to stem the flow of words or outpouring of emotion; if it does, withdraw a little and ask them to continue.

During these times you, too, may be brought to tears. This is not only normal, it also demonstrate your humanness and compassion. This becomes a catalyst for the dying person to continue with whatever it was that brought on the tears. A word of caution is necessary here – if your response is extreme or if you are inconsolable, the focus may shift from the dying person to you. The outpouring may cease, not only now but also in the future, for fear of upsetting you again. If you are unable to contain your emotions or you find the going tough, seek a friend or counsellor to talk to. This will give you an opportunity to let off steam and provide you with a safe and supportive environment in which to explore your own feelings.

I should remind you that your relative or friend, although dying, is still very much alive – thus the revised title to this second edition, *Caring for the living and the dying*. Don't feel that life and death issues must be raised every time you talk. There is more than enough happening in their life to remind them of death; the last thing they need is for others to constantly remind them of what they already know. People remain who they are even in the face of death and in the absence of pathological depression will continue to enjoy and seek normal conversation as they did before their illness. Some days they will want to talk of life and living, what is happening in the world, share a yarn or even tell a joke; at other times they may be more reflective and wish to talk about their illness and dying. Your task is to tune in, read their mind and body language and go with whatever is happening at that moment.

As the illness progresses and death nears, people's staying power diminishes and their interest in the world and things around them contracts. They may talk less and their ability to speak of the real issues may diminish. At these times, silence and non-verbal communication become more important. Sitting in silence for prolonged periods is often more meaningful than the spoken word. There may be little sharing (as we know it), but the dying person now needs your comforting presence and love more than ever. Silence is a powerful means of communicating, not only between people but also with oneself.

Guilt

Guilt may arise over almost any issue. Those who are dying may blame themselves for the pain and suffering that others experience, for the 'trouble' they are causing, for 'abandoning' their family, for not having provided for them as well as they would have liked or for failing to complete a long-promised job. They may also blame themselves for falling ill or for not responding to treatment. These regrets are normal. Unreal as they may be, the dying person needs to talk about them if only to let go of them.

Occasionally, their thoughts may become anchored on some unhappy and, until now, long-forgotten event. This may be a trivial past hurt or a wasted opportunity, but sometimes it can be more painful and invoke shame as well as guilt. There is a reluctance to talk about anything that involves guilt, but when shame accompanies guilt the reluctance and the need to talk are usually much greater. Unburdening may then assume confessional proportions as the person seeks forgiveness as well as understanding. They may struggle for weeks to let go of the thing that troubles them. Ultimately, and only with enormous courage and unending trust, they seize the occasion and reveal all. This is often followed by a profound silence and enormous relief, which may be expressed in tears or a hug.

> *The split between the way a person feels on the inside and the way she appears on the outside is usually maintained at considerable cost, with increased feelings of meaninglessness and decreased feelings of choice.*
>
> STEPHANIE DOWRICK
> *Intimacy and Solitude*

Henri Thoreau said 'The mass of men lead lives of quiet desperation'. Maybe he was right, and, if so, I wonder how many people die with years of guilt locked inside. Mick could easily have been one of these except for one precious moment.

Mick was in his late forties; he was of Eastern European background. He had come to Australia 15 years earlier. He was a loner, had few friends and his only remaining family lived overseas. He was admitted to the hospice with a diagnosis of end-stage AIDS and at the time his major complaint was constipation. Well, that is what the referring letter said but, when asked, Mick's response was 'I am full of shit'. I was taken aback by his descriptive language but assumed this meant he was indeed constipated.

Mick proved to be a real challenge. He was a very angry man and frequently abused the staff. Despite his manner I persisted in my efforts to befriend him and did everything possible to relieve his 'constipation'. Each day I would ask Mick how things were and I always got the same reply – 'I'm full of shit'.

In time I realised that Mick was not constipated. So, when I next visited, I pulled up a chair, sat beside him and said, 'Mick, tell me what you mean when you say you are full of shit'. A long silence followed. I knew something was happening and, although tempted to ask again, I remained silent. All of a sudden Mick started to sob and managed to blurt out, 'I am full of shit because I raped my younger sister before I left home'. I was stunned and

> *did not know what to say. I sat in silence as he continued to cry. I stayed with him for quite a while and, although few words were said, there was no lack of communication. Mick had, at long last, openly acknowledged his shame and freed himself from the terrible guilt that had plagued him for the past 15 years. Whether he was able to forgive himself I will never know, but he died several weeks later a much less troubled man.*

I tell this true story not because such events are common but to show the importance of trust in a caring relationship. Dying can be a very scary business, but trust and meaningful human contact give people the courage to share their good and not so good life experiences.

This element of trust is like gold for a dying person. They need to trust that the doctors, nurses and carers know what they are doing and that they will guide them through this frightening and, for them, unexplored territory. They depend on the support and encouragement of their family and friends. They need to trust these people to journey with them as far as circumstances allow. They know that they alone must make the final transition but are comforted by the knowledge they will not be abandoned, irrespective of what happens, what is said or how long the dying takes.

> *...the opposite of being in despair is believing...*
>
> S. KIERKEGAARD

Hope

That well known saying 'Hope springs eternal' says a lot about the value of hope and how we depend on it during tough times. Realistic hope is a catalyst for living. Unrealistic hope, on the other hand, leads us, as if blindfolded, down a dead-end street. The longer we travel this road the harder it is and the less time we have to retrace our steps and find the right path. Contrary to popular belief, hiding the truth rather than telling it is what undermines hope. Awareness of the truth inevitably leads to a re-evaluation of life and a reassessment of hopes. In the context of illness, it may lead to the hope for a cure being replaced by 'mini-hopes' such as the hope to remain pain-free and independent and to live as long as possible. The transition is not easy, but failing to make the shift and living in a state of denial is ultimately more harmful.

Bob was transferred to the hospice following treatment for a brain tumour. The transferring letter said he was unaware of the diagnosis as his wife and two adult children had insisted he not be told. I found it hard to believe that he was not at least suspicious that all was not well. He had a large scar on one side of his head and radiotherapy had resulted in hair loss. Despite my uneasiness, I agreed to respect their preference on the understanding I was not bound by it if Bob asked me about his condition. Reluctantly, they agreed.

For a week Bob, his family and I lived out this charade. Then one day as I was with him he asked, 'Why am I in this place?' I was both alarmed and relieved. I suggested his wife and family should be present to hear what I had to say. He rang them immediately. They rushed to the hospice and within one hour of his request we were all sitting down together. His wife sat as far away from her husband as the room allowed. The two children sat by their father as if ready to comfort him. His brother was also present.

I asked Bob to repeat his question. As I carefully and slowly explained the situation, Bob took hold of his children's hands and sought his wife's eyes across the room. She was unable to engage him. I said all that needed to be said. A tense silence followed and Bob then began to cry. At this point, his wife let go with all the hostility she could muster, blaming me for his distress. In the middle of this Bob got up from his chair, sat beside his wife and spoke quietly to her. They held each other and, as they sobbed, their two children joined them. A few days later Bob was discharged home but was readmitted and died several months later.

Some time after Bob's death I received a phone call from his brother. He told me that, following that fateful meeting, Bob had used the remaining time to deal with unfinished family matters. Bob told his family how much he loved them and did what he could to ensure that his wife, who had been unwell, would be adequately cared for after he died. My confirming what he had already suspected had freed him to do the things he considered important in his life. He fulfilled his mini-hopes.

As a palliative care doctor I am often asked by family not to tell their loved one that he/she is dying. Their reasons vary and while they attribute it to their culture and tradition, it is, more often than not, based on the belief that it would be too upsetting for the person to know. My experience has been the complete opposite. When I tell someone they are dying I only confirm what they already suspect, and rather than horror, there is a sense of relief associated with the news. Sure, it is not what they hoped to hear but it is better than living with uncertainty. There are times when truth telling is better done in little steps than in one large leap and, as with Bob, the news is best given with all the family present. Invariably, it is the dying person who copes best of all.

Dying is a journey and, if someone with a life-threatening illness is unaware they are dying, they are unable to complete many of the preparatory tasks. They may be denied the opportunity to complete unfinished business, say goodbye and have a say about where they wish to die and on funeral arrangements. In other words, they could rightly feel cheated.

Life is a constant search for truth. We grow rather than shrink from its revelations even when the truth is painful. We have an amazing capacity to incorporate the truth. The potential harm that arises when we hide from it or when it is concealed cannot be stressed too highly. Leo Tolstoy's classic, *The Death of Ivan Ilyich*, is a dramatic example of the destruction that may occur when truth is avoided. Never underestimate the strength and courage that we possess to overcome adversity, even when this involves death. Man, says Tolstoy 'has wings to lift him above the abyss'.

George had cancer of the throat and was admitted to the hospice with a severe chest infection. He knew his cancer was incurable but no one had actually told him he was dying. He was devastated when he heard this news but in reality it came as no surprise. He had wondered why he felt so unwell. Now he knew. Like all of us, George did not want to die. He said he still had a lot of living to do. When asked about this, he spoke of his only daughter's forthcoming wedding and how important it was for him to attend. Hope for cure and long-term survival had vanished but George wanted, more than anything, to see his daughter married. No guarantees were given but a promise was made to try to make this happen. Not only did George get to the wedding, he got up from his wheelchair and walked his daughter down the aisle. George completed his most important unfinished business and died shortly afterwards.

Denial

To explain the purpose of death you must study the meaning of life

FRANK HARDY

Denial is a very useful means of cushioning the effect of any shock. We resort to it frequently in life so it is not surprising to find it very much 'alive' in the context of a life-threatening illness. Denial reliably appears when a person first receive a diagnosis of cancer or some other serious illness. While it may take many forms the following statements are good examples of denial in action: 'That can't be true'; 'I will get another opinion'; 'This can't be me they're talking about'. Following the initial shock, reality ultimately sinks in and the diagnosis is acknowledged, even if not fully accepted. A mixture of hope, denial and despair characterises the treatment phase of any illness, and the way we feel is influenced by the presence or absence of symptoms, the results of tests and the messages (verbal and non-verbal) communicated by the medical profession.

When treatment fails and the person is told what they fear most – 'The cancer has come back' or 'The illness has not responded to treatment' – shock returns and is followed by any number of emotional responses, particularly depression, despair, anger, fear, resignation or any combination of these. Denial may return but it is now diluted by constant reminders and visible signs such as loss of appetite, loss of weight, altered body image, worsening fatigue and numerous other symptoms.

The determination to fight the illness, the wish to survive, fear of death and a touch of denial may at this stage drive someone to look for a cure irrespective of the cost. People seek out diets, complementary treatments, meditation, prayer or 'healing' of any form. Some go to extraordinary lengths and may travel overseas or resort to unproven and questionable treatments that drain them physically and financially. Sadly, this drive to find a cure may be under the direction of a family member whose own determination stems from their denial as much as from their suffering. Worse still, it may not be what the sick person wants, but they will do it if only to please others.

If asked about complementary therapies, my attitude is to respect a sick person's wish to explore options. I accept that these treatments may not influence the course of the illness but the measure of control they give and the ensuing journey may be more important than the outcome. The benefits of complementary therapy often appear in unexpected ways. The person may or may not feel better, disease progression may or may not slow, and death may or may not be delayed. We hope for the best but, if the best does not eventuate, the sick person and their family are more likely to accept the inevitability of death knowing that everything has been tried. Because doctors do not always see the hidden value of such a journey and because they tend to look at results and outcomes, they are not always the best people to ask when deciding on the merit of complementary treatment. More information on complementary therapies appears in Chapter 5, 'Day-to-day care'.

Judy was a young woman with a rare and aggressive form of cancer that was diagnosed during her first and only pregnancy. Because of the pregnancy she could not begin treatment until after the delivery, by which time the cancer had spread. Not surprisingly, treatment failed to slow the growth and Judy became more debilitated and eventually required oxygen for prolonged periods. She tried very hard to be a mother to her now three-year-old son but the limitations imposed on her by the cancer made this almost impossible.

One day she announced she was going overseas to see a healer who, at the time, had been in the news. I was alarmed not only by the belief that it would be a fruitless exercise but also because it would take her away from her family for several weeks. I also had major concerns for her safety. Nonetheless, Judy embarked on this journey and to everyone's surprise the whole trip went rather smoothly. On her return, however, she was no better and in constant need of oxygen.

As her breathlessness worsened, Judy found it increasingly difficult to manage at home and she was ultimately admitted to the hospice. During her stay I gathered enough courage to ask her about the overseas trip and whether she felt it was worthwhile. To my surprise she said, unhesitatingly and most sincerely, that it was the best thing she had done. I struggled to understand the meaning of her words and somewhat naively probed for an explanation, knowing she had not been cured. She looked at me and with a rather wry smile said, 'I did not go to be cured, only to be healed.'

This story led me to reconsider the meaning of the word 'healing' and how there can be such a thing when one is facing death. We are all familiar with the word 'cure', which is what others do to make someone better. It generally involves doctors doing something to the physical body such as curing infections, ulcers, migraine and so on. Healing, I came to realise, is what sick people do for themselves and, unlike a cure, it usually involves the psychological or spiritual dimension of their life. Therefore, a person may, like Judy, heal themselves yet still die. Before Judy died, I came to understand what healing meant for her. She accepted the inevitability of her death but she could not accept, and grieved over, the fact that she would lose her son, her husband and family. She also had other important unfinished business and, as a result of the pilgrimage, had not only dealt with all these matters but had also found a peace in dying that she had not considered possible before the visit. Initially, I thought she was denying her illness but I now know it was I who was denying her needs.

So denial, except in its extreme form, is a relatively common and healthy way of coping with serious illness and the prospect of an early death. I regularly see it at play in my conversations with people who are dying. After talking for some time about their illness and their impending death they may raise the topic of a holiday, which in the context of their illness seems totally unrealistic. Is this denial or is it a fantasy, and does it really matter?

I would like to believe it is human nature at work, helping that person to cope with the emotional burden of their illness and giving them something to look forward to, no matter how unlikely. It is very similar to how we fantasise about a holiday and how the thought of this keeps us going even though we may be emotionally and physically exhausted by work or other commitments.

Does it matter? If a person talks about an unlikely or unrealistic holiday but at other times talks about their dying, then it does not matter. They know they are dying and fantasising about a holiday is not a serious denial but a way of coping with grief. Very few who are dying are unaware of their fate. We will all face death in our own particular way. From an outsider's point of view, the task is not to have a plan to keep the dying person on track but to allow them to find their own way. Otherwise, their dying becomes our agenda and, thinking they are lost, we invite them to join us on our wayward journey. This is unhealthy for all concerned and particularly for the one who is dying, for in joining someone else's journey the dying person abandons their way and is less likely to be healed. Mary d'Apice in her book *Noon to Nightfall* sums this up very nicely when she says, 'You do not have to accept what people do but understand what leads them to it'.

Much more serious then is the form of denial that exists or is falsely propagated by others. Family or friends who claim that their loved one is looking better when they patently aren't, or who insist they continue diets and complementary therapies when death is nigh, do serious harm to themselves, their loved one and others who collude with them. Similar harm follows if the medical profession consciously or unconsciously engages in its own form of denial by persevering with treatment when it is not working. Truth is ubiquitous and cannot be hidden or disguised by any form of denial. No one can hide from what is deeply felt, and persevering with denial only adds to the isolation a dying person already feels. Ultimately, this proves harder to live with than the thought of death itself. Beverley McNamara, writing in *Death and Dying in Australia*, gives the following clear message:

> *The experience of each terminally ill person depends to some extent upon the resolution of uncertainties, but of course this resolution is closely linked to the nature of communication between professional hospital staff, patients, and their families.*

Ours is both a death-defying and a death-denying society and we tend to conceptualise death only as something that deprives us of life. This is epitomised by a comment made by Phillip Adams in *Death and Dying in Australia*, where he somewhat flippantly describes death as 'a full stop to the life sentence'. In some ways he is right, but only if you accept that any punctuation, including a full stop is, necessary to give meaning to any sentence. Death is what gives meaning to life and we are less likely to deny death if we do not deny its significance.

Anger

Anger, like all feelings, is a form of communication.
It brings us a message.

ELISABETH KÜBLER-ROSS AND DAVID KESSLER
Life Lessons

A dying person's anger is nearly always part of a grief reaction and is one of the hardest emotions for carers and relatives to deal with. It may be externalised and clearly visible, or internalised, when it commonly manifests as a depressed state and is therefore easily overlooked. Factors that predispose to anger or depression include the loss of control of one's life, loss of independence, and the frustration and helplessness that accompanies these and the other losses that illness brings. It may take one minor incident or a series of catastrophes to render latent anger overt, but occasionally it remains buried and then it becomes depression. The factors that trigger the anger may be real or imaginary, major or minor. Typical scenarios include reaction to things unwanted or unpleasant, things that are not done the 'right' way, disappointments, excessive noise, people 'fussing', relatives who don't visit or who visit too often, excessive pain, the failure to ease pain and so on.

Even though a particular person or incident may incite the anger, anyone becomes fair game, particularly if they happen to be in the wrong place at the wrong time. The closer your links with the dying person the more likely you are to become the target of this legitimate but misdirected anger. Remember, as the carer you are rarely the source of their anger, but you are the safest outlet for it.

When anger surfaces, give the person the time and opportunity to 'let off steam'. In keeping with the well known saying that anger generates a lot of heat but not much light, the outburst may be cathartic, but if it does not get to the source of the problem (i.e. grief) it will be revisited on more than one occasion. Attending to the incident that caused the outburst may defuse the anger but will not address the underlying problem. Anger not only clouds thinking but also hides the truth, so the chance of healing is remote while ever it persists. This is not to say that anger is bad or destructive – it may be the only emotion that wakens the dying person to their pain and ultimately opens the door for the 'deeper messages' to surface. So don't dampen, retaliate, rationalise or withdraw from a dying person's anger. It is a disguise for pain. Give them the space and security they need, stay with them physically and emotionally, and in time the anger will give way to grief. If the situation does not improve or indeed worsens, advice should be sought from the treating doctor.

The situation may be extremely testing if the anger does not resolve or is directed your way. It is hurtful to be the target of criticism, particularly when there is no basis to the assertion. You may feel unappreciated and somewhat compromised in trying to defend yourself or to respond to the accusations. There is no easy answer to this dilemma as there are so many unknowns. The golden rule of listening rather than reacting is still the safest option. If outbursts are frequent, vindictive or traumatic, seek help. Defending yourself may be counter-productive but stating your pain clearly and non-judgementally, using 'I' messages (e.g. 'I feel hurt when you speak to me that way') may just be enough to turn things around.

There will be many times when you, too, become angry. This is more likely to happen as your loved one's health deteriorates and you take on more and more responsibilities. You may feel angry with your loved one for not getting better or for the demands others place on you. Tensions may arise from the lack of perceived support from family or for unrealistic expectations they have about treatment or prognosis. Your concern for your ailing relative/friend and your helplessness at not being able to make things better may predispose you to uncharacteristic outbursts. Tiredness caused by an ever-increasing number of demands, lack of sleep and efforts to maintain some sense of normality in your life can compromise your health and also your emotional state.

Don't hesitate to tell your loved one when you feel tired, stressed or in need of a break. This level of honesty facilitates a form of communication that encourages understanding and resolution and will, in most instances, circumvent a crisis. The need for a break is not a sign of failure. Persevering when you are physically and emotionally exhausted benefits no one and may be as harmful to the one you care for as it is to yourself. Seriously ill people are very attuned to what is happening around them and it will come as no surprise when you tell them how you feel. They know what it is like to feel exhausted and will understand your need for respite. When a need such as this conflicts with your desire, take comfort in these words:

Your soul is oftentimes a battlefield, upon which
your reason and your judgement wage war
against your passion and your appetite.
Would that I could be the peacemaker in your
soul, that I might turn the discord and the
rivalry of your elements into oneness and melody.
But how shall I, unless you yourselves be also
the peacemakers, nay, the lovers of all your elements?

KAHLIL GIBRAN
The Prophet

Anger may also arise out of misunderstandings or confusion about treatment, particularly if you and your loved one get conflicting information about what should be done or when your expectations of treatment are at variance with what is happening. This is more likely when your relative is transferred from one place of care to another (e.g. from home to hospice) or if there is a sudden change in their condition or when death is very close. Good and ongoing communication by way of regular meetings involving your relative/friend, family, doctors and nurses is an effective way of preventing or dealing with these problem areas. These meetings are organised as a matter of routine when someone is admitted to a hospice or palliative care unit. They usually take place several days after the person has arrived. This gives staff enough time to get to know your relative/friend and to gain a better appreciation of the overall situation. There is, of course, no barrier to an earlier meeting if you feel that is necessary.

Joy

The discussion so far has been confined to a variety of emotions that commonly arise in those with a life-threatening illness. Individually or collectively, these emotions form part of the package we call grief and, while they are no longer seen as unavoidable milestones along the way, many or all of them may occur at some time in the course of the illness. As a carer you will be caught up in the gravity of the situation and your own responsibilities. While this is unavoidable, you can, in the process, easily overlook priceless moments of joy and happiness that also occur.

Pick up any book that specialises in grief or talk to any doctor about the subject and you will find the focus is almost exclusively on what, for want of a better word, are 'painful' emotions. I am not suggesting that grief is not painful, but wish to point out the tendency that we all have to get caught up with the darker side of grief.

In a humorous but worrying snapshot of the medical profession, Dr Marc Cohen states that medicine is obsessed with negative rather than positive mental states. He reviewed the medical literature over the past 30 years and found that 300,000 articles have been published on pain, depression and anxiety but only a mere 3,000 on pleasure, joy and happiness. This may say something about the seriousness of medical practice, but it also makes me wonder if this seriousness is reflected in the attitude doctors bring to their work and the expectation they have of those they treat. One of the real hazards faced by people who are seriously ill is the risk that their disease may overrun their life and the care they receive. If care deals only with pathology, it can result in the human spirit dying well before the body succumbs. Seeing the one you love die is hard enough, but to witness a slow erosion of the person (personality) that you knew is more painful and can lead the family to say that the person in the bed is no longer the one they knew.

Many years ago my daughter, who was eight years old at the time, said to me after an unhappy experience with an adult that the difference between adults and children is that adults forget how to have fun. Not only is this generally true, it also suggests that happiness, not sadness, is our natural state. Laughter comes more easily than tears, a smile is more common than a smirk, we naturally seek pleasure rather than pain and we find love more rewarding than hate. If we have a greater longing and natural capacity for positive emotions, surely this longing must be as great, if not greater, during times of grief? It is said that grief is a response to loss. Maybe joy needs to be added to the long list of losses.

What has this got to do with palliative care and, more specifically, with the care of your loved one? Simply this: do not be consumed by the occasion. Be aware of how easy it is to be caught up with caring and to neglect nurturing. Despite the responsibilities that go with caring, the pain and suffering that you and your loved one will endure and the sadness that hangs threateningly over your lives, there will be times of joy, happiness, excitement, awe and wonder. These moments are not manufactured, but will appear spontaneously and in some instances regularly. Quite often they arise when reminiscing about the funny, the bizarre or the unusual. Even things that were once painful are often seen in a more humorous light. When these moments arise, embrace them, enjoy them, bathe in them and do not feel guilty about the pleasure they bring. Reminiscing is an excellent way to communicate, to bridge barriers, to contact emotions and ultimately to heal. So do not hesitate to pull out photographs or show videos as a way of creating an environment for remembering.

Dying is painful and sad for all concerned but it does not exclude humour or joy and is only made worse when we miss moments of happiness or opportunities to laugh. Tears of joy are as effective in relieving pain as are tears of sadness.

...she who kisses the joy as it flies
Lives in eternity's sunrise.

WILLIAM BLAKE

Chapter 12

Your journey after caring is complete

The death of a loved one is a deep wound that heals naturally provided one does nothing to delay the healing.

PHILIPPE ARIÈS

Chapter 12

Your journey after caring is complete

Thirty three years ago our fourth child, Moira, died as a result of a cot death. Despite the intervening years I remember the day as if it was yesterday. It was 3 pm and I was sitting in my office dictating letters when my secretary put a call through from my wife, Ann. I don't know why, but I sensed something was terribly wrong. There was a brief moment when time appeared to stand still, as if to draw my attention to what was about to follow. Then, choking on her words, Ann managed to tell me that our youngest child, Moira, born just four weeks earlier, had died. Every ounce of energy drained from my body as I stared blankly at the wall ahead. There were no thoughts, no feelings, just over-whelming numbness. That moment is forever etched in my mind and memories and emotions flood back even as I write about it now.

Nothing anyone could have said would have prepared Ann or me for that moment, or for what was to follow. Our lives, our relationships with each other, our children, family, friends and colleagues were turned upside down. We felt as if an invisible force had violated us. We felt threatened by the enormity of the event and were helpless in the face of it. The control we usually maintained over our life had, in an instant, been wrested from us and we laboured through each minute of each hour of each day. Ultimately, pain replaced numbness, meaningless days followed restless nights, disturbing thoughts and unanswerable questions filled our minds and death, now unmasked, started to consume our life. We were increasingly troubled and haunted by an event we could not yet comprehend.

How you feel, behave and think following the death of someone close is unimaginable, and the experience will surprise you as much as it will pain you. There is, as grieving husband and author, N.W. Clerk said, 'a kind of invisible blanket between the world and you'. You not only lose someone you love but also a way of life and a way of being. Life is cut short 'like a dance cut in mid career or a flower with its head unluckily snapped off … so many roads once; now so many culs de sac'. This is how Clerk described his own grief after the death of his much loved wife from cancer. Author and doctor, Elizabeth Lee likens the feeling to the moment of birth where there is both agony and incredible love, and CS Lewis likens it to losing a leg – part of you is lost forever.

We are creatures of habit and the way we grieve is a reflection of how we have always coped with adversity. The loss of someone you love will have you retreating into all the familiar ways. If you have previously cried when you were upset, you will cry when you grieve. If anger, silence, caring for others or getting on with things was your habit, it will now be your crutch. Grief will have your signature all over it and will teach you more about yourself than most other things in life can. So never question why you feel a certain way or why you do or don't do certain things. 'Why' questions are only confronting and confusing. Don't disown the feelings and behaviours or try to change them but rather get to know them and experience them. They are then more likely to open and reveal a part of you that until now may have been the silent partner in your life.

I cannot be sure of how you or anyone will grieve, but the following comments reflect common responses and patterns of grief. You may recognise some part of you in there and it may throw a little light on your own grief and the journey you are now on.

What can you expect?

Grieving is a complex process and the way you grieve will be influenced by many factors, including:

- your relationship with the person who has died
- the nature and duration of that person's illness
- the coping mechanisms you usually adopt
- the length of time you had to prepare for the death
- the manner of the person's death and the amount of associated suffering
- the suddenness of the death
- any recent bereavement
- religious and spiritual beliefs
- your value system
- your culture
- other on-going stressful situations such as life event issues and personal or relationship problems.

The way your grief will unfold and the way it will affect you are totally unpredictable, but what is certain is that the intensity of the emotions that form a large part of grief will be unlike anything you have experienced before. John O'Donohue described grief in his book, *Anam Cara*, as a journey that is only a quarter inch long and several miles deep. This is not meant to imply that the grieving period is short, rather that the depth of the emotions is profound. It also suggests, correctly, that improvement is very very slow. This 'stuckness' is what makes one day seem as bad if not worse than the last. You will frequently feel all alone, as if in a deep dark hole, and wonder whether there can be any escape. Slowly, almost imperceptibly, the grief eases and you will climb out of this hole. Some sense of normality will ultimately return and the wounds will begin to heal, though not completely.

This journey you must take, the one we call 'grieving' is not out and back. You are unlikely to return to the same point at which you started. Not only does your life change: so also will you. Grief will reshape your life, your priorities, your beliefs, your attitudes and your faith. Grief induces change like nothing else you will experience. Grief takes you apart and, in putting the pieces back together, you will be different, with a changed perspective on life as well as on death. The repercussions of your loved one's death will be felt throughout the family, among friends, colleagues and perhaps the local community. Grief casts its net widely.

For some considerable time you will feel numb and act as if you are dazed – actions will be somewhat automatic. You may find yourself doing familiar things such as cooking or setting the table for two or buying food your loved one liked to eat. You may also live in expectation that he/she will walk through the door at any moment or be at the other end of a ringing phone. Long established routines will be lived out in your mind and the pain that accompanies these allows grief slowly to permeate the numbness. It is only when all the essential paperwork has been completed and most of your friends and relatives have returned to their respective worlds that the full impact of the death hits. It is then that you realise your loved one is not coming back.

Grief usually hits its peak four to eight weeks after the death. During this time and for many months after you will be on an emotional rollercoaster with many ups and downs and twists. Many of these emotions may appear in a single 24-hour period. Reminders like a favourite tune on the radio, a photograph that you recover, mail addressed to the deceased, memories of things you did together can put you in a spin, when only moments before you felt you were coping well. Do not shirk the painful memories or the reminiscing. Hiding from them does not make the pain go away or the journey any easier. It is usually better to deal with grief up-front rather than fight a continual rearguard action. The poet Rilke puts this in more symbolic terms: 'If the devils are driven away the angels will also take flight.'

How will I feel?

The duration and course of your loved one's illness will greatly influence the way you feel after they die. If there has been a lot of suffering or if the illness was prolonged, you may feel relief when death finally arrives. Relief may also be felt because the responsibility you assumed in caring for your loved one has now passed, or some unfinished business was completed before the time of death. The relative of one of my patients described this as feeling 'sadder but lighter'. There are many reasons why you may feel sad but relieved; this is absolutely normal and not an indication that you do not care.

Anger, resentment and intolerance are also very common and may be directed to the one you were caring for or to other members of the family for things they did or did not do. These emotions and any resulting conflict are almost inevitable in a caring situation and do not in any way indicate an absence of compassion or love. In fact, it is often because of love that they arise. Professor David Kissane, writing in *Death and Dying in Australia*, emphasises that feelings of resentment, conflict and love can coexist. When contradictory feelings arise, don't push them away. Acknowledge them and hold on to them in a space of love. It is the failure to recognise and own these uncomfortable feelings that causes harm. The feelings themselves are normal and often transient. It is the expectation we have of ourselves that makes them seem abnormal, keeps them alive and ultimately causes us to feel guilty.

If death follows closely after diagnosis, anger and resentment may be directed at the medical profession. This may involve their failure to effect a cure, the type of treatment your loved one did or did not receive or the medical profession's failure to inform you of the seriousness of the situation. Alternatively, you may just feel angry. There may be no particular focus for your anger – you may be angry with the whole world and with your God. Whatever the reason(s), don't harbour this emotion, bring it into the open and look at it. If a person is the object of your anger, talk to them and attempt to resolve the problem, but only when you are not consumed by anger. Aim for a win–win outcome. If anger is directed to the one who has died, talking it through with a friend or someone you feel comfortable with is helpful.

If the death involved a lifelong partner or a child it is not unusual to feel that life is not worth living. Occasionally, thoughts of suicide may be entertained. Early in my career, a reaction like that would have had me scurrying for a prescription pad or the telephone to make an urgent referral to a psychiatrist. I have since learnt that the wish not to continue living occurs in a very high proportion of those who grieve and is an expression of grief rather than a death wish. As the wife of one of my patients once said, 'It is not that I want to take my life – I just do not want to live this way'.

Suicidal thoughts spring from a deep sense of loss and talking about the loss takes courage and indicates a desire to heal the wound. The greatest risk is not with those who talk about suicide but with those who don't, or those who try to talk and are not heard. Morbid thoughts are persistent and/or intense in up to 10 per cent of the bereaved. If you fall into this category, talk to someone – it may be too tough a course to negotiate safely on your own.

Grief may also affect you in many other ways. Grief can impair your thinking and the way your body behaves. Lack of energy, aches and pains, difficulty sleeping (or excessive sleeping), loss of appetite, nausea and weight loss can often have you believing that you too are unwell. Other symptoms such as forgetfulness and an inability to concentrate may reinforce a belief that you are losing your mind.

When I was in private practice it was not uncommon for someone to visit me shortly after the death of a relative/friend with symptoms similar to those of the deceased. They feared for their own life and the convincing nature of their symptoms brought them along. More often than not these symptoms were a reflection of underlying grief, a grief that had gone unrecognised. This so-called 'somaticising' of grief occurs with both sexes but is thought to be more common among men. Men and women readily admit to physical symptoms but some rarely talk about emotions and find it hard to believe their pain and lethargy arise from unacknowledged sadness, anger or depression.

Possible repercussions

Death or even the anticipation of death has effects that can temporarily destabilise the immediate family. Each family member grieves differently, depending on their emotional as well as their familial relationship with the dying person. This, together with the altered family dynamics, can induce tensions, put strains on relationships and alter the normal process of decision making. Occasionally, family tensions or disagreements that appear after death are the smouldering remnants of discontent that first appeared during the course of the illness. According to medical anthropologist and gerontologist Andrea Sankar, many of these conflicts can be traced back to longstanding relationship struggles that have not been resolved.

Changing roles and responsibilities are to be expected before and after the death and this remodelling of the family unit can induce its own grief. Disagreements and hurts are sometimes inevitable, but the likelihood of long-term damage is reduced if family members communicate with each other, remain tolerant of each other's opinion and are prepared to negotiate. You will discover there is not one single way to grieve. As indicated earlier, the course of your grief and the strategies you use will be different from those of any other person involved. There is therefore a need for tolerance. After the death of our daughter, for example, I found myself on a completely different path from Ann and for a time that proved difficult and lonely, as we were lost to each other. This dissonance is not at all uncommon, particularly with parents who have lost a child, and may result not only in emotional separation but in physical separation also.

It is not unreasonable to expect a spouse, partner, close friend or relative to be the most supportive and understanding person in times of grief, but often they are not, only because they are struggling with their own pain. If dissonance is a problem or if the risk is high, as with the death of a child, I recommend counselling early rather than later. However, I have found that individuals and parents are often reluctant to accept counselling as they see the need for it as a failure on their part. The opposite is true. To seek help in the face of grief is a sign of strength and indicates a desire to heal.

My own inability to cry not only surprised me but made me question my own genuineness when, as a doctor, I saw how easily others cried in the face of their grief. I could not understand how someone so overwhelmed by grief was unable to cry. Guilt overtook me as I struggled to reconcile what I felt on the inside with what showed on the outside. Ultimately, tears did come, but only in the safety and privacy of our home, usually when Ann and I tried to comfort each other and make sense of what had happened. It was only then that I realised this was the way I always responded to adversity. The absence of tears said nothing about how I felt on the inside. Take heed and do not make the same mistake of measuring your grief against another or against the accepted norm.

Guilt

Guilt does not need any invitation to visit. It makes regular appearances and may have top billing in any grief story. In our case, there were many 'what ifs', 'if onlys' and 'whys' – these all exposed the guilt we both felt. We would replay the events surrounding Moira's death over and over, wondering what we had missed, what clues were overlooked and what we could have done to prevent the tragedy. As is always the case, there were no answers, just more questions and more heartache.

You too may have lingering doubts that cause you to feel guilty. These may relate to the way you cared for your loved one, negative feelings you harboured at some time, including the hope that death might come quickly. Caring for someone you love while they arc dying is extraordinarily arduous. Mistakes will occur and emotions may at times run high, but that is the norm, not the exception. I know of few if any situations where things ran without a hitch. Forgiveness, acceptance and understanding are required in large doses when you care for someone you love. You regularly shower compassion on the one who is dying and members of your own family. This is fine, but you need regular servings as well. Be gentle and kind to yourself. Be very aware of your own needs and the dangers inherent in self-recrimination, as that may become a self-fulfilling prophecy.

What a man thinks of himself, that is which determines,
or rather indicates, his fate.

HENRI THOREAU

Guilt is often more subtle and may occur at the most unexpected times. I know of a man who, many months after his wife's death, felt guilty when his sadness started to lift. He thought the sadness and longing for his wife should have lasted much longer and was deeply troubled by the change. Coping better than you expect, the first day you do not think about your deceased relative/friend, the first outing after your loved one's death, your first laugh, can all be harbingers of guilt. Ultimately, you will be able to accept the coexistence of pleasure and pain without feeling guilt, but it can be a slow learning experience.

Remember

Remember me when I am gone away,
Gone far away into the silent land;
When you can no more hold me by the hand
Nor I half turn to go yet turning stay.

Remember me when no more day by day
You tell me of our future that you planned:
Only remember me; you understand
It will be late to counsel then or pray.
Yet if you should forget me for a while
And afterwards remember, do not grieve:
For if the darkness and corruption leave
A vestige of the thoughts that once I had,
Better by far you should forget and smile
Than that you should remember and be sad.

CHRISTINA ROSSETTI 1830–94

Managing your grief

There is no simple recipe for how to grieve, but there is ample evidence to suggest the time course is shorter and the outcome better in those who express their emotions and talk about their feelings. Some find this easier than others, but it may be a lack of opportunity that influences the grieving process. Those who can express their feelings and have a large and supportive family and/or group of friends obviously do better than people who tend to bottle up their emotions and are isolated or reclusive.

There are exceptions, but some people, often men, grieve by getting on with the job and sorting out all the practical problems. If you are one of these, be aware there may be times when you hit the wall and, if you do, no amount of busyness will help you recover. Hitting the wall may be the only way your emotions can get the message through, imploring you to stop and take note of what is going on inside. It is a call to attention, informing you that all is not well and that you should take appropriate action.

Others think they are not coping if they cry or get angry. This could not be further from the truth. The ability to express emotions is the healthiest way to grieve. Talking about the way you feel and expressing emotions acts as a safety valve and prevents an excessive build-up of pressure. Shutting off this avenue of release can result in an unhealthy and possibly dangerous build-up that may manifest in other ways such as depression or ill health.

Two of the biggest problems I faced in my grief were lassitude and my reluctance to be with people. Clerk calls this 'the laziness of grief'. Getting up in the morning was a monumental task and the thought of facing another day was often overwhelming. Physical and emotional exhaustion never left me but it was the lack of motivation that made the most mundane of chores almost insurmountable. If and when I did get started, I was surprised to find how relatively easy most things were. Starting was the real problem. Once I appreciated this fact I set myself a manageable number of tasks to do each day. This routine gave some semblance of structure to an otherwise disorganised life, helped guide me through each day and prevented the endless jobs piling up. My lifelong habit of jogging was temporarily shelved but, when I did resume, I quickly came to appreciate how much this activity contributed to my recovery. I now recommend some form of daily exercise, preferably walking, to any grieving or depressed person. Regular exercise, particularly in a natural setting, has a profound healing effect on body and spirit. It frees the mind, allowing deeper wisdom and intuitive knowledge to break through the barriers we construct to protect ourselves during times of grief.

Returning to work or resuming your 'normal' life may be another hurdle to contend with. The physical and emotional effort this involves, or the assumption made by others that you must be 'better', can make this a testing time. Returning to 'public' life exposes you to one of the most seemingly benign but difficult situations you are likely to encounter after your loved one's death. Responding to the questions 'How are you?' or 'How are you coping?' can be very confronting. I certainly came to dread this form of greeting. I was uncertain whether it was just part of the routine social engagement or whether the inquirer really wanted to know. In my case, a truthful answer was generally ruled out because circumstances were not conducive to honesty or because I did not have the emotional stamina to unburden myself once again. So I learnt to dodge the question with a nod or a shrug. Eventually, I needed to confront some friends who, through pity or genuine concern, would ask the same question several times a day as though they expected me to fall apart at any moment.

Unfortunately, grieving people are also open game for gratuitous advice. This is rarely helpful. The worst piece of advice I received was that I should return to work as soon as possible because it would help me to forget. After all these years those words still grate, and at the time they wounded me deeply. I certainly wanted to feel normal and was prepared to do whatever it took, but I did not want to forget. I had so little to remember of Moira's short life I wanted to hang onto every morsel of memory, no matter how painful. Shrouding grief with an early return to work was not going to aid my healing and is unlikely to benefit you.

Returning to 'normal' life was equally hard for Ann. She was relatively isolated at home, but it was the isolation she felt as people crossed the street or changed direction when they saw her coming that was painful and made her feel like a modern-day leper. Fortunately, there were also those who went out of their way to be with her. The most helpful were those who listened and heard her distress. For those who do not know what to say or are fearful of saying the wrong thing, a touch or an embrace is all that is required to show you care.

Anniversaries, birthdays, Christmas and other significant dates can reawaken grief even if the death occurred years earlier. The intensity of the emotions after such a long time may surprise you and it is often best to anticipate these occasions and decide in advance how you wish to spend the day. You may choose to be alone or alternatively have someone special with you. Whatever you do, do not ignore the meaning and significance of these times.

Finally, choose carefully and be selective about whom you talk to. Grieving people need someone who will listen rather than give advice.

Those that give advice are unconsciously putting their own agenda before yours and may only add to your uncertainty and confusion. The painstaking work of grief cannot be short-circuited but talking about how you feel makes the journey less lonely. The best person to talk to is someone you trust and who is not uncomfortable if you fall apart. Protect yourself from unnecessary hurt by avoiding people you do not want to see and not doing things you do not want to do.

Take care not to neglect the basic necessities of life. Sleeping patterns change and appetite is frequently reduced or lost altogether. Try to maintain your usual time of going to bed. The nights may seem long and you may feel as though you do not sleep. You may only remember the periods of restlessness but, sleep will come, often in snatches. This is better than no sleep at all, and maintaining some form of routine for going to bed and rising is more likely to see you settle back into a relatively normal sleep pattern. A bedside radio, tapes or CDs can be a comfort during the long dark hours. Hot milk prior to bed may assist sleep, whereas tannin-rich teas and coffee are counter-productive, as is the long-term use of sleeping tablets.

Food may be the last thing you feel like. This may be a product of your grief or a remnant of bad eating habits cultivated while you were caring for your loved one. Food, like sleep, is essential for your body. Physical and emotional healing can be impaired by the lack of either, or both. Try to cultivate a regular pattern of three meals a day. Small servings are less likely to be rejected than large meals. Don't eat on the run and, if there are others in the house, try to sit down together. Cooking (and the associated shopping) may be one of many chores you cannot face in the early phase of your grief. Have friends cook and do other practical things for you. This not only relieves you of chores but gives others a simple and useful way of being with you.

Caregiving is physically and emotionally demanding so don't be too surprised by the consequences. Exhaustion and a whole gamut of emotions will accompany you for longer than you can imagine.

How long will I grieve?

This is a question you will ask of yourself, especially when times are tough or when grieving goes on longer than you had imagined. There is no answer, nor any way to predict. Living with the expectation that 'this' must end soon is normal but unhelpful and will ultimately sabotage the normal grieving process. The answer is the old but familiar story of taking one day at a time. Just as water finds its own course following a torrential downpour so too does the flow of emotion that accompanies grief; any attempt to block or redirect the flow will only lead to a greater outpouring once the levy breaks. As unlikely as it may seem at the start, life will at some time in the future take shape and a sense of normality will slowly return. This process may take months or years.

Those who express their grief fare better in the short and long term than those who bottle up their feelings. If you find this hard, pull out old photographs, play favourite music and visit places that hold fond memories. These are good ways to release emotions that may have settled but still weigh heavily.

Grief is an uncomfortable and unpleasant state to be in but it is unavoidable if someone you love dies. Healing and moving on in life is not possible without it. Relatives and friends may not see it this way and may suggest you shake yourself out of it, try to forget, go on a holiday or return to work. Such comments often reveal their discomfort and desire to have you feeling better. Do what you choose to do and not what others say. You are extremely vulnerable at this time and can do without unhelpful suggestions. If, on the other hand, you choose to take a holiday or return to work, that is okay, but it is good to talk this through this with someone you trust only because either move can sometimes introduce new or unexpected complications.

Several weeks after Moira's death we went to stay with Ann's family in New Zealand. This removed us from the ever present memories and we were greatly assisted by the love and support we got from caring relatives. The two weeks' respite was just what we needed and we thought we were all the better for it. When we returned home we were shocked to discover how quickly the grief returned. We were right back into the rawness of what we had left behind. That was a shock and we were not prepared for it.

Finally, it is suggested that any major life decisions should be delayed and not made early in the course of grief. Stability rather than change is essential at this time. Contemplate change by all means, include all those who will be most affected by the change in your discussions, but make haste slowly.

Communicating with family

Your verbal and non-verbal communication is important when other family members, particularly children, are involved. You may not be able to help each other but to isolate yourself because you are in pain, or because you do not wish to upset one another, creates gulfs in a relationship that can be misinterpreted as not caring. Your partner, spouse and children may feel sidelined by your isolation and uncertain how best to help. Just to say you feel lousy today, or that you need space or a hug, fills the gaps that can otherwise be misinterpreted. Communication is a two-way process, so remember to check how others are and give them plenty of hugs in return. They too are hurting.

Kids are extremely intuitive and can sense when things are not right. They know their life has been disrupted but, depending on their age, they may not always associate this with the death. Their confusion is further complicated by all the resulting changes within the household, the loss of security and seeing people they love cry, possibly for the first time. One of the commonest ways they manifest this confusion is through changes in behaviour. So be understanding and give them plenty of time. Tell them how you feel and how much you love them. Explain why things are different, why familiar routines have been broken and why there are lots of visitors. Listen to their concerns, answer their questions and feel their unique form of pain. If you do not include them in your grief they may blame themselves for the way you feel and may even hold themselves responsible for the death.

Our daughters, who were aged five and three when Moira died, told us some years later they were confused by all the activity and emotional turmoil but what disturbed them most was the sight of their parents crying. This was new to them and as frightening as Moira's death itself. They also feared her death might have been a result of something they had or hadn't done. One of them was guilt-stricken and believed that putting her dirty fingers into Moira's mouth might have caused her death. Not surprisingly, she was too afraid to talk about it at the time. The lesson to be learnt is that kids can read much more into the situation and into our grief than we could ever imagine. The only way you will know is by listening to them.

Children can move quickly between the sadness of death and the fun of childhood. They may be full of sorrow one minute but playful the next. Our five-year-old, though very sad, hoped Moira's death would not interfere with her birthday party, which had been planned for a few days later. Such ambivalence is common and very normal in children, as it is in adults. Ann and I were surprised by this and many other things, but came to realise how obtuse and pervasive a child's grief can be. Our two daughters, Claire and Ruth, would cry, but usually in concert with us, not because they were sad but, seeing both of us cry, they felt they should keep us company. Our other child, James, was almost two and, while he does not remember the occasion, I have vivid memories of him repeatedly entering Moira's room after she had died as if wondering what had become of her. His confusion was painfully obvious even if it was not stated. David was born 15 months after Moira died but even he was not immune to the effects of her death. In his formative years he often asked if he was a replacement for Moira. He needed lots of love and reassurance before he was able to accept his own inherent worth. See Chapter 8 for more information on how to communicate with grieving children.

Complicated or protracted grief

On occasions grief is complicated and protracted. This is often a result of the circumstances surrounding the death but can occasionally stem from a relationship that binds the grieving person to the one that has died and prevents them from moving on. Complicated grief has nothing to do with the intensity of emotions; problems are more likely to arise (but not always) with those who do not show emotion. Similarly, there is no time limit on how long one grieves; what is important is how grief affects a person's life and whether it becomes a barrier to them readjusting to life without the deceased.

There is no single feature that identifies complicated grief but severe or prolonged physical neglect is probably the most obvious. Refusing to eat over a considerable period of time, marked weight loss and excessive use of alcohol and/or drugs may be telltale signs. Serious mental distress, uncharacteristic or unusual behaviour, persistent morbid thoughts and disturbed thinking are more serious and may indicate a need for medical or psychological help. Counselling is now available as a Medicare benefit so cost should not be the barrier it once was.

The following list is not exhaustive but in the context of a life-threatening illness, it describes circumstances that may predispose a person to protracted grief. Grief that results from or is complicated by any of these may require extra support from family and friends as well as professional help, regardless of whether any of the above warning signs are present.

- Sudden, unexpected death
- Suicide
- Death in which considerable pain and suffering was involved
- Death of a child or young person
- Death of a young mother/father
- A series of deaths
- Social isolation following the death of someone close

- An elderly person widowed after a long and happy marriage
- Financial hardship

Suicide is uncommon among those who grieve, but it is not unusual or abnormal to feel that life is not worth living or to contemplate suicide. If you have morbid thoughts and cannot be certain of your intentions seek help from someone you trust. Ring Lifeline (see Appendix) or some other grief support service or see your doctor. This is a difficult step to take when you are so depressed but asking for help is the first and most important step in the process of healing. To be able to say 'I am frightened', 'I am scared', 'I am depressed' takes enormous courage but sharing this with someone you trust, even someone anonymous such as a telephone counselling service, can be a huge relief. This unburdening and letting go of your grief is what heals.

Your concern about the emotional state of someone else who is grieving can also be a tricky situation. No one wants to overreact but neither do you want to overlook possible warning signs. If you are a close friend or relative of the person, share your concerns with them honestly and compassionately. They are unlikely to be upset by your concern and may in fact be grateful and relieved. Rather than making the situation worse, it may provide the opportunity they have been waiting for but have been too afraid to create for themselves. If you don't feel comfortable about doing this, discuss the situation with the person's next of kin or your family doctor.

Unusual events

One of the most common but least recognised aspects of grief is the so-called 'paranormal' phenomenon. This somewhat mysterious term refers to events or experiences that are out of the ordinary and for which there is no plausible explanation. In the context of grief these experiences may include one or more of the following:

- extremely vivid dreams in which the deceased appears and brings some form of message
- visions of the deceased
- the impression that the deceased is beside you
- hearing the deceased's voice
- a sense that you are being touched by the deceased
- smelling her perfume or his aftershave
- an unusual happening such as a clock stopping, a picture falling from the wall or a flickering light, just as you speak of the deceased.

These experiences are common and absolutely normal in people who are grieving. If you experience anything like this, rest assured you are NOT going mad. The American Psychiatric Association has recognised these experiences as part of the normal grieving process. Many studies have shown that up to 40 per cent of those who grieve have at least one of these experiences within the first few months of their bereavement. Some may have many more, but this is the exception rather than the rule. The most common experience is the sense of the deceased person being present in the room, but vivid dreams or hearing the deceased's voice are also reported frequently. People say these experiences feel absolutely real and, although initially frightening, the experience becomes something they treasure.

I have had some people ask why they have not had any of these experiences when others have. Widows, particularly, felt a deep sense of hurt and wondered why they had missed out. We simply do not know why these experiences occur with some but not all. It is too big a question for us to understand and to suggest otherwise assumes we know what happens after death. The only reassurance I can offer is that failure to have one of these experiences often means that everything that needed to be said was said before the time of death.

The phenomenon itself has intrigued many researchers and begs the question as to whether these experiences are a form of hallucination or evidence for life after death. No proof exists either way. For me, the question of cause is academic and will never be resolved. What is important is the significance and the meaning people attach to these experiences. Although messages are rarely given, most say they 'know' what it is all about. They can describe the events quite clearly but the understanding is more of an intuitive knowing. It is something that is sensed rather than heard. This may sound nebulous to the outsider but it is as real as it is indescribable for the one who has the experience.

If you have one of these experiences, treasure it and be reassured you are not going mad. You may wish to keep it to yourself, but sharing it could be helpful. If you do, choose someone you trust, someone who will listen and who will validate you and what you describe.

Many years ago I was the palliative care doctor for 'Red'. As the name suggests he had a shock of red hair which, by the time I met him, was thinning through age and ill health. He had a large cancer involving the side of his face and, despite pain and the need for daily dressings, he did his best to maintain a normal life. This included frequent fishing holidays with his wife and three daughters, one of whom had recently married a man of Italian descent. Red loved the outdoors and, despite his rapidly growing cancer, he and his family spent their last Christmas camped on a river bank. The only thing Red loved more than fishing was his family, who in turn showered him with understanding, love and care.

During one of his hospital visits Red admitted he was not afraid of death but was worried about who would do all the repairs and practical things after he died. He had been a very practical person throughout life and this concern was real for him, as it is with many men facing the same fate. Red died several weeks after his last camping holiday. The family knew that holiday was likely to be his last so they all accompanied him for those few days while he fished his favourite spot, yarned to long-time fishing mates and said goodbye to all those familiar and treasured things.

A week after his death I was contacted by his wife who wanted to tell me about something unusual that had happened. Shortly after Red's death, her son-in-law had got up from bed in the early hours of the morning. As he walked down the hall he saw Red, as clear as day, standing in front of him. He was stunned and remained frozen to the spot. He was unsure how long the vision lasted but suspects it was brief. Nothing was said but he was absolutely certain about the message Red delivered: 'You are the only man in this family. I want you to look after my wife and daughters.' The experience was so real and the message so clear his son-in-law had no doubt about its reality.

Chapter 13

Practical matters to ponder

Begin with the possible;
Begin with one step.
There is always a limit,
You cannot do more than you can.
If you try to do too much,
You will do nothing.

GURDJIEFF

Chapter 13

Practical matters to ponder

Caring for someone who is dying can be a time-consuming and energy-sapping business. Managing issues on a day-to-day basis is often the only way to cope and the thought of making plans for funerals or completing paperwork may be low on the priority list. If you have tried to get your loved one's affairs in order you may have found it all too surreal to continue, or the information may be hard to access or too confusing to process. I suspect anyone in the position of carer looks for reasons not to proceed with these confronting yet necessary issues when there are so many other care-related matters that have to be attended to. Added to this are the natural concerns of how and when to raise the subject of a funeral with someone who is dying. Will it upset them and take away whatever hope they have? Is it worth the associated trauma? This is upsetting business, a series of problems you could well do without.

In this chapter I will touch on issues that are best addressed before the time of death and some matters that pertain to the death. Experience has shown that it is better to complete necessary business earlier rather than later, but selecting the right time will always remain a challenge. The list that follows may seem daunting but, if you begin with the easiest or most urgent task and slowly work your way through, it is not so overwhelming. Seek assistance when you need it and delegate chores if you have neither the time nor the inclination. As Gurdjieff says: 'You cannot do more than you can'!

The legal status of many of the matters discussed varies from state to state. For a more complete review, I refer you to the excellent book by Stella Tarakson, *What to Do When Someone Dies* (see Bibliography).

Funeral arrangements

Planning the funeral is one of the most traumatic things to be done when someone is dying. It could be interpreted as the final step in acknowledging the inevitability of your loved one's death and, for this reason alone, many defer making the necessary arrangements until it is too late to involve the one who should have the most say. Some believe it may upset them or that it will be seen as giving up. Dying people are very aware of their predicament and are not afraid of talking about funerals – they are often relieved to have the matter dealt with and out of the way. Instead of being traumatic it can be a cathartic and healing experience, providing an ideal opportunity for the dying person to reflect on their life and talk about things they have already contemplated.

A funeral is an occasion when the bereaved farewell and celebrate the life of the one who has died. It is also a statement about that person's life. If the dying person has the opportunity to plan their own funeral, it can be their final gift to those who are left behind. If you believe this, as I do, the opportunity to plan our own funeral is as much a right as it is a necessity. So, put planning a funeral high on the priority list, do it while the person is able to participate actively, take plenty of time and do it in an environment suited to the occasion.

Choice of funeral director

All funeral directors stick to a code of conduct and are governed by the same rules, so the choice of director is usually based on practical matters such as cost and location. Reputation and other people's recommendation are sometimes useful guides. If you are unsure, visit some of the funeral directors in your vicinity before making a choice. This is one chore you could delegate to a close family member who has the time, for it could be somewhat traumatic. Remember to discuss your thoughts with your loved one before making a final decision. Once that decision has been made, tell the funeral director of your decision, record the name and phone number and keep this information with other important contacts. The next contact you have with the funeral director will be when you phone to inform them of your loved one's death.

Burial or cremation

Some people have strong views on burial and cremation while others have no particular preference. Again, it is important for your loved one to have a say but costs, circumstances, customs and beliefs will determine the ultimate choice. Any funeral director can provide information that may assist you in reaching a final decision.

Special needs

If there is a cultural or religious practice or ritual you wish to observe at and around death, ensure the information is conveyed to people that may be affected, such as nurses, doctors and the funeral director. These wishes and any associated requests should be recorded and a copy given to those involved in caring for your loved one.

Keeping the body at home

There is now not only a move towards people dying at home but also towards keeping the body of the loved one at home for as long as possible after death. This was once limited by law to eight hours following death but the legislation has been relaxed and now permits a body to be retained at home for up to five days. In special circumstances the Director-General may approve a body being retained for a longer period. If you choose to keep your loved one's body at home for any length of time, notify the funeral director earlier rather than later. He/she will then advise you on the optimum environment that should be maintained within the home after death.

Irrespective of the length of time you keep your deceased relative at home, remember to turn off all heating in the room, including electric blankets, and remove all warm bed covers as heat will speed up the post-mortem changes. It is also important to contact the nurses promptly so they can wash and lay out the body before stiffness (rigor mortis) sets in. You may, of course, choose to do this yourself or you may feel more at ease assisting the nurses. For further information on what to do after death, see Chapter 7, 'What happens around the time of death'.

Home viewing

A home viewing immediately prior to burial or cremation is something that can be arranged through the funeral director. It gives the family an opportunity to have a private farewell immediately before the more public funeral. Some think this is a great idea but others are concerned that the presence of a dead body in the house may create unhappy associations, particularly for younger members of the family.

Post-mortem

A post-mortem is rarely required when death is not unexpected and there are no suspicious circumstances. If the circumstances of death are not clear, or if the person dies within twenty-four hours of surgery or a general anaesthetic, or if a doctor has not seen the deceased during the last three months of life, the coroner must be notified by the attending doctor. A post-mortem is then mandatory. If someone has a life-threatening illness but dies suddenly or sooner than expected, and none of the above conditions apply, a post-mortem is not required by law.

Sometimes a post-mortem may be requested by the treating doctors, not out of any legal requirement but to clarify some unusual aspect of the illness. This can be a real dilemma if the request comes out of the blue and has not been discussed prior to your loved one's death. If that is the case, you should obtain as much information as possible about the reasons for the post-mortem and ask what exactly will be done and what, if any, tissues will be removed. Ask for time to think about it and particularly to discuss the matter with other family members. Ultimately, you must do what you are comfortable with, bearing in mind how your relative/friend may have felt about the procedure. If you agree to the request you will have to sign the necessary paperwork, which should include any special requests or restrictions you place on the examination. A post-mortem should not delay or interfere with the funeral arrangements and the funeral director will take the body of your loved one to and from the place where the post-mortem is to be performed.

Organ donation

The suitability of your loved one's organs for donation will depend on their age and the cause of death. Rarely are organs suitable for transplantation if the person is aged or has died of cancer or some other chronic illness. The only exception to this is the cornea (the covering over the coloured part of the eye). These can be donated irrespective of age or condition; even those with widespread cancer can donate corneas if they so choose. If you or your loved one requires further information on organ donation your doctor will advise you or put you in contact with the appropriate organisations.

Death certificate

Following the death of your loved one, a death certificate and, if required, a cremation certificate will be completed by the local or hospital doctor. An official copy of the death certificate will be required to complete outstanding financial and legal matters. This cannot be supplied immediately and is only available from the Registry of Births, Deaths and Marriages in your state or territory (see Appendix). Applications are usually made through the funeral director. They will complete the application form and forward it, together with the death certificate and all other information required to register the death. A fee of $44–$65 applies, and the copy of the death certificate is usually available within three working days of application. The next of kin, the deceased's solicitor or the executor of the will can also make application by phoning or visiting the website of the appropriate registry. Unofficial copies may, of course, be obtained by making or asking for a photocopy of the original certicicate(s).

Who needs to be notified after death?

Many agencies will have to be notified of your loved one's death. The funeral director can provide you with a list of the usual government contacts but there may be others. When you are speaking to your loved one about funeral arrangements, ask if there are any special friends, colleagues or associates that they would like notified after death. Some of the more important commercial agencies include:

- Centrelink
- the bank or other financial institution

- life and other insurance companies
- superannuation funds
- Medicare
- the Roads and Traffic Authority
- the Australian Taxation Office
- the Electoral Office
- credit card operators.

Pensions and allowances

Illness can be a very expensive business. Medical and pharmaceutical costs pile up while financial reserves slowly evaporate. You may be one of the many people in a caring situation unaware of the financial help that is available via a carer's allowance or disability pension. If you are linked in with a palliative care service, ask to speak to their social worker. They can advise you on these and other sources of potential income, help you to complete the necessary paperwork and fast-track their processing. Alternatively, you can visit your nearest Centrelink office and discuss your situation with them.

Wills

You hardly need to be reminded of the importance of a will, but I wish to stress the value of preparing it well in advance. Like many practical issues, the matter of a will is often deferred until the very last moment for fear of upsetting the dying person. In my experience this is rarely the case – it is often something the person wishes to finalise, if only to move on to other important business. It can also be a moving and meaningful experience as they decide which personal item they would like to leave to whom. Contentious issues can also arise and the earlier these are dealt with the better.

Most people have wills in place before illness becomes a reality. If the will is reasonably current and circumstances have not significantly altered there is probably no need to update it. If circumstances have changed and you are concerned the will could be contested, seek legal advice. As with all things, the earlier this is done the better – the closer someone is to death the less energy and inclination they have to deal with contentious issues. Confusion is also more common as death nears and this may render the person incapable of making a legally binding will.

When confusion is present and doubt exists about the person's competence to make a legally binding will, a doctor is asked to determine their capacity to understand the nature and ramifications of the decisions they may make. The doctor also needs to be assured that all decisions are made freely and without duress. As confusion is often an intermittent or reversible problem, capacity may vary from day to day. If a person is incapable of making a legal will one day the situation should be kept under review and, if there is any improvement, the doctor can be asked to reassess the situation.

Enduring Power of Attorney

An Enduring Power of Attorney is a legal document that gives powers to an appropriately appointed person to make and enact financial decisions on behalf of someone sick or dying. This power comes into effect only if the person making the appointment loses capacity, and it ceases at the time of their death. The advantages of having a trusted person manage financial affairs and carry out transactions in this situation is obvious. The appointment can only be made if both parties understand fully the nature of the power and what sort of things can be done. The sooner an Enduring Power of Attorney is made the better, as the problem of confusion could interfere with its implementation.

Three practical points are worth noting.

1. An Enduring Power of Attorney requires a solicitor, barrister or clerk of petty sessions to explain the nature of the appointment and

to ensure all parties understand and agree with the appointment. The solicitor then witnesses the necessary completion of the certificate.

2. An Enduring Power of Attorney made in one state may not be recognised in another.
3. To act appropriately, the appointed person should be familiar with the contents of the deceased's will. For this reason, it is usually the next of kin or a close relative/friend who is appointed.

Enduring Guardianship

An Enduring Guardianship is a piece of legislation that exists in some states and territories and allows for the appointment of a person to make legally binding lifestyle decisions for someone, should they lose the capacity to do so. This covers:

- where the person should live
- what health care services they should receive
- what medical and dental treatment they should receive.

As with the Power of Attorney, the Enduring Guardianship only comes into effect when the person making the appointment loses the capacity to make their own decisions. The Enduring Guardianship ceases when the said person dies. There are restrictions as to who can be appointed as Guardian and, for obvious reasons, anyone involved directly in the medical care of the person making the appointment (e.g. a doctor or nurse) is excluded. You, as carer and/or next of kin, are not excluded and would be eminently suitable to fulfil this role.

The Enduring Guardianship is a powerful and useful piece of legislation. It acts as an advance directive, allowing the appointed Guardian to make legally binding decisions on behalf of the dying person on matters of treatment and care. It also means that doctors are unable to give treatment a Guardian does not consent to. On the other hand, doctors may refuse to give treatment if they disagree with the Guardian's recommendation. The appointment of a Guardian is one way of ensuring that a person receives the type of care they want at and around the time of death. From a carer's point of view (subject to your being appointed Guardian), you continue to have an important and legally endorsed role in the way your loved one is treated, provided the decisions you make fulfil the directives recorded by your loved one on the Guardianship form.

Both the Enduring Power of Attorney and Enduring Guardianship are legally binding documents. They ensure that the dying person maintains control over their financial situation and the way they are cared for around the time of death. Once the documents have been completed, make sure they are accessible and available when needed.

Advance Directive *(see also Chapter 9)*

With medical science's increasing ability to keep sick and dying people alive, many people seek to ensure that their existence will not be prolonged by treatment or technology when there is little or no hope of a meaningful recovery. Instead, they seek an assurance that they will be kept pain-free and their death will be dignified. In an attempt to guarantee this, Advance Directives have become a popular means of stating one's wishes. Victoria, South Australia, Queensland, the Australian Capital Territory and the Northern Territory have legislation that provides for Advance Directives. While the other states do not have similar legislation, Advance Directives may still be valid under common law (see Bibliography – Biegler, P). To ensure its legal status the directive should be current and completed in accordance with the recommendations. The directives must be reasonable and consistent with acceptable standards of medical practice.

Like an Enduring Guardianship, an Advance Directive is particularly useful in the face of unexpected illness or injury, especially where the person may be unable to give clear directions about their treatment preferences.

The Department of Health in most states and territories has literature available on Advance Care Directives and Enduring Guardianships that will help you in your choice and the legal completion of the documentation. Whatever you choose, pay detailed attention to the wording of the document, as ambiguous or vague statements can be challenged. Legal guidance is recommended and is indeed necessary with the Enduring Power of Attorney and the Enduring Guardianship.

Chapter 14

Steve's story

Love of oneself and self-forgiveness are prerequisites for dying well.

Chapter 14

Steve's story

Your experience in caring for someone you love and being with them as they die brings you face to face with the reality and mystery of death. In this book I have sought to deal honestly and pragmatically with the events and emotions that accompany death but, in so doing, the mystery that surrounds such an occasion becomes inescapable. The metaphysical dimensions of death and the shifts people make as they die have been highlighted in many of the stories, raising questions for us all.

The story of Steve's final twelve months of life illustrates the potential for change and the importance of time in allowing these changes to permeate the 'excesses' that accumulate throughout life. Steve's life and death had a profound and lasting effect on me. My entrenched views and preconceived ideas were blown away during those twelve months and left me to wonder at the potential that lies within us all.

Steve was in his early thirties when he was admitted to hospital, having suddenly and for no obvious reason become paraplegic. After many tests the doctors informed him he had a rare cancer of the spine that was inoperable and also incurable. It was a death sentence, but Steve had received a fair share of body blows in his short life and he brushed it off. He greeted the news with a string of choice Australian expletives and insisted on being discharged back to his home, a single room in a large boarding house where others like him sheltered from life.

Steve was no ordinary 33-year-old. He had spent most of his adult life bouncing between boys' homes, mental institutions and jail and had moved to Sydney not to start a new life but to continue the old in a setting where he was less well known. He carried with him many labels – psychopath, schizophrenic, hard-nosed criminal, dropout, misfit. He was not a very nice person.

At the boarding house the owners did all they could to make Steve comfortable but the responsibility of caring for him in that setting was beyond them. They insisted on outside help and, despite his objections, palliative care nurses were called in to assist with his treatment and day-to-day care. The nurses were emotionally and physically strong and had successfully managed many trying patients in the past, but they had never come across anyone like Steve. He was difficult, lacked all social graces, had a foul tongue and resisted all efforts to keep him clean. Despite this, fellow guests at the boarding house cared for him, ran his messages, placed his bets and kept him company. In return, he treated them with as much respect as he was capable of.

Out of frustration and concern for his welfare the nurses asked me to visit him. They thought he might listen to another man, a doctor and an authority figure. How wrong they were! I had done my homework and imagined how I would approach the situation. The manager of the boarding house pointed to Steve's room but then disappeared. I thought that was strange. I knocked on the door and, hearing a grunt, tentatively entered the room. Steve was stretched out in bed, naked except for a sheet covering the lower part of his body; a cigarette hung from his mouth and the bedside radio was loudly broadcasting a race meeting. I was about to introduce myself when Steve lashed out – 'Who the f... are you and what the f... do you want?'

I had not expected a warm welcome but I had not anticipated this. Somewhat unconvincingly I said, 'I am Michael, the palliative care doctor.' As I was to learn later, Steve could read a person and a situation in a flash. He knew he had the upper hand and was determined to drive home the advantage, but he also needed to check my staying power. He said, 'Can't you f...ing see I'm busy, you'll have to come back some other time.' Grateful for the opportunity to leave and take stock of the situation, I asked if the same time tomorrow would be okay. I took the audible grunt to mean 'yes' and left the room.

The next day I went back. 'It's me again,' I said, as I knocked and slowly opened the door. He was less hostile and, in between orders to people in other rooms and orders for me to open windows then close windows, he gave the impression of listening to what I had to say and he even allowed me to examine parts of his damaged body. But he remained defiant and refused to allow the nurses to do any of the things I recommended.

Several weeks passed and eventually I received the call I had been dreading. The nurses said things were getting out of hand, Steve's problems were worse and they were helpless to do anything about them. 'Could you admit him to the palliative care unit for a short time to see if that makes a difference?' I immediately had visions of Steve swearing, smoking and bossing everyone around and wondered how the staff and the other patients would cope. I tried desperately to think of alternatives but none came to mind and, after a meeting with the staff to prepare them for what could only be a torrid time, I arranged for Steve to be admitted.

My fears were well founded. Within five minutes of his admission Steve had offended most of the nurses, the cleaning and kitchen staff, as well as the unfortunate man who shared his room. Among his many orders were repeated demands that he be allowed to smoke in his room. Regulations had never stopped him in the past. After a hurried meeting with senior staff, we sat down with Steve and tried to work out some ground rules that might make life bearable for us all. He listed his demands, which included his need to smoke, place bets and have regular lashings of 'junk' food. In return we asked for cooperation with the nursing and medical care he was to receive, and at least an attempt to stop swearing. We arranged for him to be wheeled outside to a shaded area to smoke, and for volunteers and others to do his essential shopping.

The road was rocky but after one month it was clear we were making some progress. Steve hardly swore and when he did it was followed by an immediate 'Oh, s…, I'm sorry'. He and his room-mate became close friends and when the man died Steve was visibly upset and found it hard to conceal his tears.

Being a chain smoker, Steve spent more time out of his room than in it. The palliative care unit had a designated outdoor smoking area. It was a nice protected spot, though it lacked a view. Tall, suffering pot plants made up for the concrete surrounds. The area was large enough to take Steve's bed and still leave ample room for other smokers to gather round. And gather they did. Steve became a popular figure with his fellow patients and also their friends and relatives. He was a great entertainer and a good listener and could immediately recognise when someone was in pain or needed to talk. In a strange sort of way, Steve became our de facto counsellor. He knew what it was like to suffer and could relate to those who were troubled. Visitors would often spend as much time with Steve as with their relative/friend and many of them returned to the unit after the death of their relative, just to see Steve.

In the first few months of his stay Steve often asked to go home. Home to his friends at the boarding house who, incidentally, continued to visit right up to the time he died. I'm not sure whether Steve really did want to go home or whether he thought that going home would be a sign that things were getting better. We tried, but something always cropped up to stop the plan. If it wasn't pain or some other problem, it was the lack of a suitable room. Eventually, Steve stopped asking and I suspect it was because he knew he was not going to get better.

Steve was a great one for talking about his feats but never about himself, his family or his 'pain'. Then all of a sudden the floodgates opened and, not only did he talk, he insisted that it be recorded as he was sure it would bring him fame and fortune. He wanted someone to listen and record his story by hand rather than put it on tape and the reason soon became obvious. An elderly Irish Catholic volunteer (whom I will call Patricia) had befriended him and they had formed a wonderful relationship. She became a mother figure to him and he loved and respected her as he did his biological mother. Patricia came several days a week and recorded his sometimes horrific story verbatim. Her only proviso was that he refrain from the colourful language that invariably appeared as he became excited or agitated. When Patricia was not there others filled in, and I was one of the regular scribes. I could hardly believe some of the things he said but convinced myself that, if they were not fact, they were metaphors for his life and not lies.

After several weeks of non-stop talking, Steve started to withdraw and became overtly depressed. What started off as tales of bravado gradually changed to stories about home and family. Stirring up the past had brought more to the surface than he had bargained for. He began to have recurrent dreams of someone trying to slay him with a knife and these were so vivid and real that he was afraid to sleep at night. He used every ploy he knew to stay awake and it was not uncommon to see Steve in the smoking area at all hours of the night, smoking or eating or chatting to the night staff. He talked about his fear of dying and for the first time started to cry.

He wanted to see his parents, who'd been in regular phone contact but had not yet visited. They lived interstate, but now they began to visit regularly and this was the start of a healing process for Steve. I don't know what they talked about but it was clear their visits meant a lot to Steve. He started to glow, but his body was wasting quickly. The tumour was quite massive and the pain was obviously bad, but the only time he complained was when the fear of dying overwhelmed him.

By now Steve held almost celebrity status within the palliative care unit. A party planned for his birthday had to be held in an adjoining building that had a room large enough to house the masses. Family, staff, patients and visitors joined in the celebration. Steve received more gifts on that one birthday than he'd had for the previous ten years. As he lay, confined to bed, surrounded by people, smiling his anything but Colgate smile, opening gifts, talking without swearing, I reminisced about that initial visit many months earlier. I wondered how many more people there were like Steve, who just want to feel loved and valued.

Steve's tumour had grown to such a size it was pressing on nerves and other painful structures. As a result he could neither lie flat nor sit upright. Only a few positions gave him brief periods of comfort. Despite this, he collared me one day and said he had not been to the beach for years and would like to see one before he got too sick. How sick do you have to get, was my immediate thought. But his enthusiasm was childlike so I spoke to the nurses, volunteers and ambulance officers and they all thought it was a great idea. They organised ambulance transport and an accompanying crew, made up of Patricia, one other volunteer and myself.

They made the long trip to Maroubra (20–30 kilometres) and I arranged to meet them there. Steve and his entourage duly arrived. His pale, gaunt face was painted with sunscreen and he wore an ill-fitting hat. The ambulance officer wheeled him onto the concourse and found a shady spot where Steve could look at the surf and the few board riders. It was a beautiful day but I had little time to soak up the scenery as Steve had me trotting to the local shops. He ate very little but insisted we savour the delights of Pluto Pups and Dim Sims. Patricia sat by him except for a brief time when Steve released her so that she and the other volunteer could walk along the promenade. Steve enjoyed the outing but pain and discomfort limited his stay to just over an hour. He did not complain of pain but simply said he would like to go back to 'his bed'.

Steve had completed all that he needed to do. He was at peace with the world, his family and most of all he was at peace with himself. The layers of anger, bitterness, hatred and disregard had peeled away to reveal a vulnerable, frightened, compassionate human being, still with faults, but faults he could now recognise and no longer needed to defend. As wasted as he was, it was another three months before Steve died. His funeral service was held in the same room as his birthday with just as many people present. But instead of laughter there were tears and instead of bearing gifts we gathered to acknowledge the gifts Steve had given us all. Steve had completed a journey I would have thought impossible – indeed, it may not have happened had he not had as much time as he did.

Lead us into the darkness that we may find what lies concealed.

MICHAEL LEUNIG
The Prayer Tree

What is unusual about Steve's story is the length of time he had, after diagnosis, to contemplate his life before he died. One year is a long time to be dying. Many people live longer with a life-threatening diagnosis, but, unlike Steve, they often create distractions that temporarily relegate dying to the background. Steve had no distractions – no surgery or chemotherapy, no diets or complementary therapies and no one to search for miracle cures. Steve contemplated death in a way described by Leo Tolstoy in *The Death of Ivan Ilych*: 'It [death] drew his attention to itself not in order to make him take some action but simply that he might look at it, look at it straight in the face...' Steve did not want to look at death but it was always there, in the form of pain and paralysis, or in thoughts that he initially dared not confront. When these failed to draw his attention, death appeared through the medium of dreams and from these there was no escape. The dreams told Steve in no uncertain terms what he already knew, but had resisted.

Steve confronted his beasts and died a different person from the one who had entered the unit twelve months earlier. We are told, 'people die the way they have lived.' Steve may seem to contradict this but the fact is that people, including Steve, do not change because they are dying: we simply see another side of them, not something new but something newly revealed. The situation is analogous to Michelangelo's comment about the magnificent sculptures he created. He said that beauty was already present within the stone and that all he did was remove the excess. Dying removes the excess that accumulates through life and reveals only what is already there. This indisputable fact underpins much of the healing that is possible when someone is dying. As they come to know this part of themselves, free of the excesses, the invisible thread that held their life together becomes visible, often for the very first time. To discover there is a pattern to life, no matter how disconnected or dysfunctional that life may have been, is often the catalyst for healing and is responsible for what is otherwise seen as change. Removing the excess may afford the dying person the first opportunity to understand who they really are. This form of self-discovery is not only liberating; it also often leads to acceptance and self-forgiveness, the basic requirements for unconditional love. Love for oneself and self-forgiveness are prerequisites for 'dying well'.

For what is it to die but to stand naked in the wind
and to melt into the sun?

KAHLIL GIBRAN

As a palliative care physician, one of my greatest concerns is that people with life-threatening illnesses in the 21st century will not have enough time to contemplate their life and to heal whatever needs to be healed. The cure imperative has become so strong and the belief in medicine so great, society now believes that many of today's illnesses are curable and, for those that are not, life can be prolonged through the marvels of medical science.

Medicine has grown enormously in stature over the past twenty years, but we all still die; my fear is that medicine's plans for the future push death further and further into the background. In failing to recognise the inevitability of death, it turns a blind eye to human suffering and deludes itself into believing that death is without meaning. Death is unwelcome, particularly when it creeps up on us, surprising us like some figure emerging from the dark. But it is never without meaning. What meaning does life have if death is meaningless?

There is an enormous body of knowledge and literature about death. Of the many messages that come through, none stands out more than the words of Scott Peck: 'When we shy away from death, the ever-changing nature of things, we inevitably shy away from life'. This reinforces the strong, close relationship between life and death, a relationship that has always existed but is increasingly neglected or denied in a world that attempts to redefine life at the expense of death. There can be no life without death or death without life – together they complete the cycle of life. Not surprisingly, then, preparing for death teaches us about life and helps us to lead a more fulfilling life. Laying claim to the fact that we will all one day die is what makes life as valuable as any treasure, and death the treasure chest that contains it.

Dying is one of the most important times in a person's life. Preparing for it means leading a full and good life, as best we can. To reflect on this life as it draws to an end is what brings completion. To relive all that has been beautiful or painful, to talk about relationships that have been replenishing and those that need healing, to face our beasts, to speak of the people we love and to remember the wondrous things that have blessed our life. The most peaceful people I have seen die were those who, like Steve, had time to do all these things. The first step in this journey is the hardest and takes courage. However, in the words of the ancient sage Lao-tzu, a journey of over 1000 miles begins with one step.

If we can accept death as part of life, not just as the end to life, living and dying become inseparable. Rather than a shadow that hovers over life, death becomes the light that illuminates the way of life. Death, according to Marie de Hennezel, psychologist and author of the book *Intimate Death*, 'can be the culmination of a shaping of a human being'.

Epilogue to second edition

I must seek to embrace insecurity
as one of the essential marks of our humanity
and strive to help people understand
that it is no longer a vice, but a doorway
into a new understanding of our humanity.

JOHN SHELBY SPONG
Eternal Life

Recently I cared for an elderly man as he was dying of cancer. Communication was difficult as he had a tracheostomy – a tube in his windpipe to assist with breathing. As a result, our conversations were as laboured as his breathing, for his only means of communication was with pencil and paper. Despite this, Joe always wanted to 'talk', sometimes about the pain he experienced, but more often about his distress at not being able to die. I was not surprised at this. It is not an uncommon feeling among the elderly, particularly those burdened with an incurable illness.

After several weeks of slow and deliberate conversations, Joe finally told me about a recurrent dream which clearly disturbed him. In this dream, he would see the faces of fallen war comrades. These were mates he had fought with in World War 2, but who did not, like him, survive to return home. Joe cried as he attempted to put down the story. His tears and the tremor in his writing hand were clear evidence of the grief that still gripped him after all these years, yet he needed to write all this down for me to read. When he had finished, we sat together, him crying and me wondering what I could do other than hold him by the arm. After a little while I said something like, 'war is a terrible thing', and he replied, 'so is guilt'. I did not know what he meant and asked for clarification. After some time it became clear. Joe felt guilty for being the only one of his company to survive the war. Almost seventy years ago he had wanted to die with his mates; and now, he was still alive and unable to die despite an extensive cancer involving his throat and neck.

Over the following weeks we talked about the dream and Joe's guilt at surviving the war. The dream continued, but his interpretation of it changed. He now saw his mates as waiting for him and he looked forward to meeting up with them again. Joe was a widower. He had two grown children whom he loved, and they him, but he was ready to move on and wondered what he had to do to for this to happen. Joe died several weeks later. He was, by this time, more at peace with himself. I would like to think he died after he was able to resolve and finally let go of the guilt he had carried over all these years. He no longer feared meeting up with his mates – he was looking forward to a reunion.

Death is a strange thing. We know it is inescapable – Woody Allen, in his inimitable way, says, and I quote him a second time, 'no one gets out of this world alive'. What continues to surprise me, however, is the path each of us takes as we are dying. It is clearly different for every person, but there is something common to each and every journey.

Metaphorically speaking, death holds a mirror by which those who are dying see back into their past and recapture and relive many of the meaningful events that have permeated their life. Interpreting and understanding these experiences is often the challenge. William Wordsworth refers to these experiences as 'spots of time'. They are the vital links in a chain of events that constitute life. It is these vital links that are likely to surface as death nears – links that need to be processed and their value recognised. The memories we have of these experiences may be happy or not so happy. There may be joy, but often there is fear, anger, guilt or remorse. Given the right environment and the best of care, however, some light is always present at the end of every dark tunnel. As carers you can create an environment where this can happen. Your presence, your love and your willingness to listen will give your loved one the courage they need to complete their healing journey. This journey may be marked by insecurity and uncertainty, but we should never forget there are also gifts to be had for both the living and the dying. To care for someone who is dying is truly a 'doorway into a new understanding of our humanity.'

My work and experiences, like that of Joe's, have led me to reflect on the nature of death and what, if anything, awaits us after death. Many of my dying patients console themselves with the belief they will meet up with friends or loved ones and this belief is often re-enforced by a dream or a vision in which they see the one(s) they hope or expect to meet. This vision or dream is not only accompanied by peace and sometimes joy, but also the certainty that the meeting will take place. What awaits us is, of course, beyond our comprehension and while I too have a yearning to meet with my departed loved ones, particularly our daughter Moira, I concur with Bishop Spong who says, '[we] step beyond words at this point into a wonder of a wordless reality.' Death is truly one of life's greatest mysteries. I do not know if there is life after death, but I do know there is life before death, and it is the quality of that life that will determine the quality of our death.

MICHAEL BARBATO

Appendix

Palliative Care Associations

National
www.palliativecare.org.au
Ph 02 6232 4433

New South Wales
www.palliativecarensw.org.au
Ph 02 9206 2094

Victoria
www.pallcarevic.asn.au
Ph 03 9662 9644

Tasmania
www.tas.palliativecare.org.au
Ph 03 6285 2514

Queensland
www.palliativecareqld.org.au
Ph 1800 660 055

South Australia
www.pallcare.asn.au
Ph 1800 660 055

Western Australia
www.palliativecarewa.asn.au
Ph 1300 551 704

Australian Capital Territory
www.pallcareact.org.au
Ph 02 6273 9606

Northern Territory
www.nt.palliativecare.org.au

Aged Carer

Information for those caring for aging relatives
www.agedcarer.com.au
Ph 0414 214 636

Alzheimer's Australia

www.alzheimers.org.au
Ph 1800 100 50

Carers Australia

Provides a range of information, resources and support to carers
www.carersaustralia.com.au
Ph 1800 242 636

Centrelink

www.centrelink.gov.au.
Ph 13 23 00

Compassionate Friends

Support service for bereaved parents, grandparents and siblings
www.thecompassionatefriends.org.au

NSW	02 9290 2355
VIC	1800 641 091
QLD	07 3254 2657
SA	08 8351 0344
WA	1800 628 118

ACT 02 6286 6134
TAS 03 6261 4250

Dementia Care Australia

www.dementiacareaustralia.com
Ph 03 9727 2744

Kidney Health Australia

www.kidney.org.au
Ph 1800 4 543 639

Kids Helpline

Counselling service for kids 5–18 years
Ph 1800 551 800

Leukaemia Foundation

(For leukaemia and lymphoma)
www.leukaemia.org.au
Ph 1800 620 420

Lifeline

Telephone counselling service
Ph 13 11 14

Motor Neuron Disease (MND) Australia

www.mndaust.asn.au
Ph 1800 777 175

National Heart Foundation

www.heartfoundation.org.au
Ph 1300 362 787

National Institute of Neurological Disorders and Stroke

An excellent US website that provides information on all neurological conditions
www.ninds.nih.gov

National Stroke Foundation

www.strokefoundation.com.au
Ph 1800 787 653

The Australian Lung Foundation

www.lungfoundation.com.au
Ph 1800 654 301

The Registry of Births, Deaths and Marriages

NSW 1300 655 236
ACT 02 6207 3000
VIC 1300 369 367
TAS 1300 135 513
QLD 1300 366 430
SA 08 8204 9599
WA 1300 305 021
NT 08 8999 6119

Bibliography

Albom M. *Tuesdays with Morrie.* Sydney: Hodder, 1998.

Bailey LW and Yates J. *The Near-Death Experience.* New York: Routledge, 1996.

Barbato M. Bispectral index monitoring in unconscious palliative care patients. *Journal of Palliative Care*, 2001;17(2): 102–108.

Barbato M. *Reflections of a Setting Sun.* Sydney: Griffin Press, 2009.

Barks C. *The Essential Rumi.* San Francisco: HarperCollins, 1995.

Barrett W. *Death Bed Visions.* Wellingborough, Northamptonshire: Aquarian Press, 1986.

Biegler P. Determining the validity of advance directives. *Medical Journal of Australia,* 2000;172: 545–548

Boden C. *Who will I be when I die.* Melbourne, Victoria: HarperCollins,1998.

Callahan D. *Pursuing a Peaceful Death.* Hastings Centre Report, 1993; 23(4): 33–38.

Clerk NW. *A Grief Observed.* London: Faber & Faber, 1961.

Cohen M. *Australian Family Physician.* 2001; 30(1): 17–19.

Cole R. *Mission of Love.* Melbourne: Lothian, 1999.

Collett M. *At Home with Dying—A Zen Hospice Approach.* Boston: Shambhala, 1999.

d'Apice M. *Noon to Nightfall.* Burwood, Victoria: Collins Dove, 1989.

Darling D. *After Life.* London: Fourth Estate Ltd, 1995.

Dass R. *Death is not an Outrage.* Colorado: Sounds True Recordings, 1992.

Dass R and Gorman P. *How Can I Help?* New York: Borzoi, 1985.

De Hennezel M. *Intimate Death.* London: Warner Books, 1997.

Dowrick S. *Intimacy and Solitude.* Melbourne: Heinemann, 1991.

Frankl V. *Man's Search for Meaning.* Boston: Beacon Press, 1959.

Fromm E. *The Art of Loving.* London: Unwin Books, 1957.

Gibran K. *The Prophet.* London: Heinemann, 1979.

Grof S. *Books of the Dead.* London: Thames & Hudson, 1994.

Grof S. *The Cosmic Game.* Melbourne: Hill of Content, 1998.

Hinton J. *Dying.* Middlesex: Penguin, 1967.

Housden M. *Hannah's Gift.* London: HarperCollins, 2002.

Jones GC. *Magnanimous Despair.* Mount Nebo, Qld: Boombana, 1998.

Jouvet M. *The Paradox of Sleep.* London: The MIT Press, 1999.

Kazan A. *Reflections on Dying.* Sydney: private publication, 1999.

Kearney M. *Mortally Wounded.* Dublin: Marino Books, 1996.

Kellehear A. *Death and Dying in Australia.* Melbourne: Oxford University Press, 2000.

Kellehear A. *Eternity and Me.* Melbourne: Hill of Content, 2000.

Kessler D. *The Rights of the Dying.* New York: HarperCollins, 1997.

Kübler-Ross E. *On Death and Dying.* London: Tavistock Publications, 1970.

Kübler-Ross E. *To Live Until We Say Goodbye.* London: Prentice Hall, 1978.

Kübler-Ross E. *On Children and Death.* New York: Collier Books, 1983.

Kübler-Ross E and Kessler D. *Life Lessons.* New York: Scribner, 2000.

Lamerton R. *Care of the Dying.* Middlesex: Penguin, 1980.

Lee EA. *A Good Death.* Old Noarlunga, South Australia: Stirling Press, 1996.

Leunig M. *Common Prayer Collection.* North Blackburn, Victoria: Collins Dove, 1991.

Levine S. *Who Dies.* New York: Doubleday, 1982.

Levine S. *Healing into Life and Death.* New York: Doubleday, 1987.

Lowentahl R. *Cancer—What to do about it.* Melbourne: Lothian, 1996.

McKissock M and McKissock D. *Coping with Grief.* Sydney: ABC Books, 1985.

May R. *Man's Search for Himself.* New York: Delta, 1973.

May R. *Freedom and Destiny.* New York: WW Norton, 1981.

Merikle PM and Daneman M.

'Memory for unconsciously perceived events: evidence from anaesthetised patients.' in *Consciousness and Cognition.* 1996; 5(4): 526–541.

Mindell A. *Coma—Key to Awakening.* Boston: Shambhala, 1989.

Moore T. *Care of the Soul.* New York: HarperCollins, 1992.

Noll P. *In the Face of Death.* New York: Viking, 1989.

Nuland S. *How We Die.* London: Chatto and Windus Ltd, 1993.

O'Donohue J. *Anam Cara.* Sydney: Bantam, 1999.

Osis K and Haraldsson E. *At the Hour of Our Death.* Norwalk, Connecticut: Hastings House, 1977.

Rando T. *How To Go On Living When Someone You Love Dies.* Lexington: Bantam Books, 1991.

Reanney D. *The Death of Forever.* London: Souvenir Press, 1995.

Remen RN. *Kitchen Table Wisdom.* Sydney: Pan Macmillan, 1996.

Reoch R. *Dying Well.* Sydney: Hodder & Stoughton, 1997.

Rinpoche S. *The Tibetan Book of Living and Dying.* Sydney: Random House, 1992.

Sankar A. *Dying at Home.* London: The Johns Hopkins University Press, 1991.

Shelby Spong J. *Eternal Life: a new vision.* Sydney: HarperCollins, 2009.

Stedeford A. *Facing Death.* Oxford: Heinemann, 1984.

Stephenson JS. *Death, Grief and Mourning.* New York: Free Press, 1985.

Sutherland C. *Within the Light.* Sydney: Bantam Books, 1993.

Sutherland C. *Children of the Light.* Sydney: Bantam Books, 1995.

Tarakson S. *What to Do When Someone Dies.* Marrickville NSW: Choice Books, 2001.

Tobin DT. *Peaceful Dying.* New York: Perseus Books, 1999.

Tolstoy L. *The Death of Ivan Ilyich.* London: Penguin Books, 1960.

Wilber K. *Grace and Grit.* Melbourne: Collins Dove, 1991.

Zukav G. *The Seat of the Soul.* London: Rider, 1990.

Index

Page numbers in bold print refer to main entries